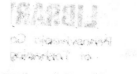
"**If you are having problems getting pregnant, Fern Reiss's** *Infertility Diet* **is a great place to begin.**" - *Dr. Alan Penzias, Boston IVF and Harvard Medical School*

"*The Infertility Diet* **provides a compelling review of the numerous links that have been found between diet and reproductive function. I'm going to recommend** *The Infertility Diet* **to my patients.**" - *Dr. Martin Keltz, Director of Reproductive Endocrinology and Infertility, Columbia University St. Luke's-Roosevelt Hospital Center, NY*

"**It is important to recognize that the dietary strategies and lifestyle modifications in this book, if applied for a lifetime, may contribute to substantial benefits in preventing hypertension and heart diseases which are leading causes of death in both men and women.**" - *Dr. Christopher O'Donnell, cardiologist, Harvard Medical School*

"**The average cost of fertility treatments is about $8,000 per attempt. The success rate is under twenty percent.**" - *The Center for Disease Control*

Peanut Butter and Jelly Press
P. O. Box 239
Newton, MA 02459-0002
phone/fax: (617)630-0945
www.infertilitydiet.com
info@infertilitydiet.com
SAN 299-7444

Printed in the United States of America.

The information herein is solely intended for educational purposes and is not intended to substitute for medical advice. The author and publisher are not responsible for use of the information in this book. Before making any dietary changes, see your doctor.

Library of Congress Cataloging-in-Publication Data
Reiss, Fern
The infertility diet : get pregnant and prevent miscarriage / by
Fern Reiss
p. cm.
Includes bibliographical references and index.
ISBN 1-893290-39-5
1. Infertility, Female—Diet therapy—Recipes. 2. Infertility,
Female—Nutritional aspects. 3. Fertility, Human—Nutritional aspects.
4 Human reproduction—Nutritional aspects. I. Title.
RG201.R425   1999   98-48227
618.1'780654--dc21   CIP

The Infertility Diet

Get Pregnant and Prevent Miscarriage

by

Fern Reiss

Special Thanks To...

The many doctors, nutritionists, and fertility specialists who read and helped this book; in particular, Dr. Alan Penzias, of Boston IVF and Harvard Medical School, Dr. Martin Keltz, Director of Reproductive Endocrinology and Infertility at Columbia University's St. Luke's-Roosevelt Hospital Center in New York, and Dr. Christopher O'Donnell of Harvard Medical School, for their endorsements; to Dr. Miriam Blum for her thorough technical review of the manuscript; to Wendy Esko and the Kushi Institute for Macrobiotic Studies; to the gang at the Culinary Institute of America; to Abby Wyschogrod for designing my website; to Dr. Miriam Keltz, Elisheva Urbas, Barb Harris, and Dr. Eric Lichter, for their time and kind referrals. To all the many friends who listened, especially Aviva Bock and Susan Schoenberg.

To my children, Benjamin and Daniel Yedidya, who are so much fun to spend time with that this book didn't go nearly as quickly as it might have. And to my husband Jonathan, for endless hours of proofing, computer help, great ideas, and especially for all his love and support, always.

Contents

Dr. Alan Penzias
Boston IVF and Harvard Medical School

If we in the medical profession had all of the answers, this book would not be necessary. As a specialist in Reproductive Endocrinology and Infertility, I sit across from couples every day trying to diagnose and treat the causes of their infertility. Despite apparently normal results to a battery of tests, many couples still face the frustrating diagnosis of unexplained infertility. Many of them will benefit from medical therapies but each couple needs to start somewhere.

We already know that there are medical benefits to be gained from a healthy diet. The prevalence of diseases such as cancer and heart disease have been altered by diet, so why not infertility? My grandmother has always felt that her chicken soup with noodles had healing powers; who knew that it was really a steaming amalgam of carotenoids, bioflavonoids, and complex carbohydrates?

If you are having problems getting pregnant, be proactive: See your doctor and start getting healthy. Fern Reiss's **The Infertility Diet: Get Pregnant and Prevent Miscarriage** is a great place to begin.

Dr. Martin Keltz
Director of Reproductive Endocrinology and Infertility at Columbia University's St. Luke's - Roosevelt Hospital Center

Fern Reiss' **The Infertility Diet: Get Pregnant and Prevent Miscarriage** offers a nutritious approach to self empowerment in the battle against subfertility. A diet based on whole foods, rich in vegetables, fruits, and grains, will reduce your risk of heart disease, may enhance your fertility, and will start you on a healthy diet in pregnancy.

The Infertility Diet: Get Pregnant and Prevent Miscarriage provides a compelling review of the numerous links that have been found between diet and reproductive function. Diet alone cannot replace the accurate diagnosis, honest prognosis, and array of treatment options offered by a reproductive endocrinologist. Yet, so many of my patients want to know what lifestyle changes they can make to increase their odds. I'm going to recommend **The Infertility Diet** as part of their recipe for success.

We Couldn't Get Pregnant

For three years, my husband Jonathan and I struggled with infertility and miscarriage. We already had one child; we were anxious to have more. But although we started trying to conceive again soon after the birth of our first child, we failed miserably. The first few months we were calm and confident. By the end, we were frantic and desperate. How was it, we wondered, that we had conceived so quickly once, and were having such a difficult time now?

Although technically the term "infertile" applies to any couple that has been unsuccessful in conceiving a child after twelve months of trying, infertility wasn't a word we liked to use, and we were reluctant to seek medical treatment. After all, we reasoned, we weren't "really" infertile—we had one child—and one miscarriage—to prove it. Still, we couldn't seem to get pregnant again.

All around us, we heard people bemoaning their infertility. All the people we knew, it seemed, were spending their time making the rounds of infertility clinics. Our friends found these experiences painful, humiliating, expensive, and depressing. Some were getting daily injections; others were attempting in vitro fertilization; still others had given up and registered for adoption. We weren't sure where we'd find the money, time, or emotional energy to jump into the fray.

When I attended a friend's baby shower I realized just how widespread the problem was. In a room of 26 women, only two had more than one child; everyone else was trying desperately for a first, or second, child. It was hard to be happy for the expectant mother when we were all waging our own battles with infertility.

The turning point for me and my husband came when I started to realize how many of our medical problems, over the years, we had solved with dietary changes and natural therapies. Plagued with a bad back since my first pregnancy, I had mostly healed myself by practicing Iyengar yoga. Diagnosed with extremely high cholesterol, my husband had stabilized his numbers by altering his diet. We wondered if there might not be a natural remedy or nutritional solution for infertility, too.

We had tried some of the old wives' tales already—a full list of these is included in Appendix A. Now we were ready for a more serious, comprehensive look at the subject. I began to sift through the hundreds of medical studies conducted in the past five years that examined fertility and miscarriage and their relation to diet.

What I discovered is that both infertility and miscarriage are strongly linked to vitamin and nutritional deficiencies. Study after study, anecdote after anecdote, reinforced this point. If that were really true, we should be able to cure it by remedying our diet to incorporate the missing foods. Though the information was scanty and hard to find, I finally succeeded in putting together a list of foods that were linked to increased fertility and miscarriage prevention.

We altered our diets immediately. We conceived two months later.

Since then, we have suggested our diet to friends and family. Many couples have tried it—and gone on to conceive.

It is certain that this plan will not work for everyone. However, since the foods are all healthy, and most have been found to help prevent other ailments such as cancer and heart disease, the worst that can happen is that you will cultivate a better diet and improve your general health. But if you are in the majority whose infertility is caused by something that might be affected nutritionally—or if doctors tell you that clinically there is no medical reason why you can not conceive—there is a good chance that an altered diet will dramatically improve your odds.

We wish you luck.

Can Foods Affect Fertility and Miscarriage?

Infertility threatens to be the epidemic of the 21st century. An astonishing one in two couples in their forties is infertile. Even for younger couples, one in five is infertile. This is an alarming increase over past years.

No one is sure exactly why infertility is on the rise. Some researchers claim that treatment is only today being sought for a malady that in past generations remained a "hidden" problem. Others point to the rising age of couples attempting to conceive. Still other researchers attribute it to environmental pollutants of all sorts.

What is clear is that the problem is real, and measurable: The average sperm count has decreased by 30 percent since 1950. Miscarriage rates, too, are high; conservative estimates claim that 25% of all pregnancies result in miscarriage; other researchers assert that including the number of women who didn't realize they were pregnant brings the number up to an alarming 70%.   And people who suspect that they are infertile, after a year or more of trying to conceive, or who have miscarried, have few places to turn.

Modern medicine can solve some infertility and miscarriage woes. Women whose infertility stems from endometriosis, for example, can become fertile once their growths are surgically removed. Other problems are harder to diagnose. Infertility tests can be inaccurate; fertility drugs can be expensive, unpleasant, and ineffective.   While assisted reproductive technologies such as in vitro fertilization (IVF) and gamete intrafallopian transfer (GIFT) increase the likelihood that a woman will conceive, the success rate even for these very expensive programs is less than 20 percent, according to the Center for Disease Control.

Many couples, after extensive medical testing, are told that there is no medical problem that should prevent them from conceiving or carrying to term—and yet they can not. Frustrated, they are ready to try anything—if only their doctors would tell them what to try!

Medical doctors, however, partly because of their generally limited training in nutrition, are unlikely to suggest dietary changes as a tool for fertility enhancement and miscarriage prevention. Yet over the last few years, the healing properties of food have received a lot of press. Everyone knows that vitamin C prevents scurvy, and that calcium helps build strong bones. And recently, scientists have zeroed in on a small list of foods they now believe can help prevent, and heal, disease. Even the FDA has finally jumped on the antioxidant bandwagon; and all across the country people are crunching cruciferous vegetables to ward off cancer.

If what you eat affects whether you will contract cancer, or whether you are putting yourself at risk for heart disease, then why wouldn't your diet affect your fertility, or your ability to carry a pregnancy to term? Certainly there is reason to believe that what you eat affects your reproductive abilities, at least in broad terms: Famine victims, for example, are unlikely to conceive. And everyone has heard about how too much coffee can lead to miscarriage.

No one has yet done extensive research on how diets that have been linked to heart attack, stroke, and cancer prevention might also combat infertility and help prevent miscarriage. A fully tested infertility diet would require many years to complete. Additionally, the government is reluctant to fund studies that do not concentrate on a single change in diet, so after a comprehensive five year study, there would be proof that only a single ingredient worked.   Thus, currently the mainstream medical establishment does not promote nutritional therapy to couples suffering from infertility.

However, although no one has conducted a long-term medical study on a complete diet, many foods have been studied in isolation.   Several hundred medical studies in the past five years have begun to establish a promising link between nutrition and fertility.

According to the Journal of the American Medical Association, diets for various ailments such as breast cancer are now being formulated by evidence-based nutritional analysis; that is, "integrating current best evidence."   The same technique can be used to formulate a fertility enhancement and miscarriage prevention diet. By integrating all the latest research, it is possible to devise a "best guess" diet that is based on a sound analysis of current nutritional research.   **The Infertility Diet** is the result of an evidence-based nutritional analysis of several hundred medical studies that explored connections between diet, fertility, and miscarriage.   It is a "best guess" diet based on everything we currently know about nutrition and its role in enhancing fertility and preventing miscarriage.

These nutritional suggestions will not work for everyone, in the same way that cutting down on fat consumption will not definitively prevent you from contracting breast cancer.   Some causes of infertility and miscarriage simply do not seem to be affected by diet. Nonetheless, all of the recommended foods are healthy, inexpensive, and easily found and prepared.

Moreover, the foods recommended on this diet are foods that have been linked to the *prevention of other diseases*. At worst, then, this diet may lessen your chances of contracting cancer, stroke, or heart disease, and improve your overall health and vitality. At best, the dietary changes may enhance your fertility, and result in your ability to conceive, and carry to term.

Finally, simply the empowerment engendered by taking part of the fertility process into your own hands, via nutritional changes, might positively affect that fertility.

For couples who have been trying unsuccessfully to become pregnant, or who have experienced the trauma of miscarriage, nutritional changes are definitely worth a try.

What Can Go Wrong and How Diet Can Help

In order to truly understand how diet can contribute to fertility enhancement and miscarriage prevention, we must first look at the normal process of pregnancy, and the many factors that must work together to ensure conception and a viable birth. By then examining some of the difficulties and problems, we can discover situations where nutritional additions and avoidances may have an impact.

On day one of a woman's cycle, the hypothalamus, a part of the brain, sends the hormone GNRH (gonadotropin releasing hormone) to the pituitary gland. The effect of receiving the

GNRH stimulates the pituitary gland to release follicle stimulating hormone (FSH). Follicle stimulating hormone then stimulates the maturation of between 15 to 20 eggs in each ovary; each egg lies within its own follicle. (One of these follicles will become the largest, or dominant follicle, and that is the one which will later release its egg in ovulation.)

If GNRH is not received by the pituitary gland—or if the level of follicle stimulating hormone released by the pituitary gland is insufficient—the ovaries' follicles will not develop properly, and there will be no pregnancy. However, there are dietary ways to assist the level of follicle stimulating hormone, and help enable the follicles to develop.

The follicles all produce estrogen, which inhibits further production of follicle stimulating hormone by the pituitary gland. Estrogen performs several tasks in the pregnancy: It stimulates the uterus to create a suitable lining (endometrium) for the egg; it causes the cervix to begin making sperm-receptive fluid; and it opens up the cervix, so that the sperm can enter.

If not enough estrogen is present in the woman's system, the uterine lining will not be prepared properly to support a pregnancy; the cervical fluid will be too hostile to the sperm to allow fertilization to occur; and the cervix will not open enough to permit entry to the sperm. However, all of these effects can be encouraged by nutritional choices that will help to ensure the production of sufficient estrogen.

When the estrogen buildup reaches a certain level, it again triggers the brain's hypothalamus to release GNRH, which then triggers the pituitary gland to release a surge of luteinizing hormone (LH). Within a day, this surge of luteinizing hormone causes the dominant follicle to burst through the ovarian wall, and ovulation occurs: An egg is released into a fallopian tube. (The other eggs that were growing disintegrate.)

If the surge of luteinizing hormone is insufficient, then ovulation will not occur. If ovulation does not occur then no pregnancy is possible. If there is a surge in the levels of the hormone prolactin (possibly the result of a common problem of a prolactin-microadenoma, a tiny, benign tumor in the pituitary gland), then the elevated prolactin levels will impede ovulation. Many women can promote ovulation by altering their diet.

The egg must be fertilized in the fallopian tube within 12 hours after ovulation for a viable pregnancy to continue. Thousands of sperm chemically adhere to the covering of the egg before one sperm fuses to its nucleus.

If the man's sperm count is low; or if a high percentage of the sperm have an inadequate morphology, or shape; or if the motility, or speed of the sperm is slow; or if vaginal conditions were too acidic for the sperm to survive, then the chances of fertilization are reduced. However, there are foods that can increase sperm count, and improve sperm morphology and motility, and nutritional ways to neutralize the acidity of the vagina.

Once the egg has been released from the ovary, the ruptured follicle, left on the ovarian wall, becomes known as the corpus luteum, and produces progesterone. (The corpus luteum will live and continue to produce progesterone for 12 to 16 days, if fertilization does not occur.   It will continue to produce progesterone beyond that only if pregnancy hormone Human Chorionic Gonadotropin (HCG) is released. (More on this later.) Progesterone thickens and softens the endometrium (uterine lining) so that the egg can implant and be nourished. Progesterone (and corresponding decreased estrogen) also dry up the cervical fluid, and close the cervix, to prevent more sperm from entering. Finally, progesterone stops the release of other eggs.

For women with a short luteal phase (less than ten days is considered inadequate), the corpus luteum does not produce enough progesterone, causing the lining to shed early (menstruation). There are, however, dietary ways of balancing estrogen-progesterone levels, and of regulating the luteal phase.

Finally, once the egg is fertilized, it will travel for several days to the uterine lining, where it will burrow in. As soon as that happens, the egg releases HCG which tells the corpus luteum to continue releasing progesterone so that the egg will continue to have a nourishing endometrium. (If there is no pregnancy, no HCG will be released; the sudden plunge in progesterone will cause the endometrium to disintegrate over the next five days in menstruation, and will also cause the renewed production of follicle stimulating hormone by the pituitary gland to start the cycle anew.)

Improper diet can lead to excess levels of the hormone prostaglandin. This can impair the functioning of the corpus luteum, causing it to produce amounts of progesterone insufficient to sustain the endometrium. However diet can correct this malfunctioning of the corpus luteum, compensating for the effect of excess prostaglandin.

A variety of other maladies, explained later—ranging from candida albicans to hypothyroidism, from endometriosis to recurrent miscarriage—can affect fertility negatively, endangering the possibility of successful pregnancy.

These, too, can be benefited by dietary changes.

Eating for Fertility: Where to Begin

In the following pages, we will discuss various foods that you should eat—and other foods that you should avoid—in order to enhance your fertility. To begin with, let us examine a few general principles.

First, this book is not organized primarily by malady or fertility problem, although you can use it that way. There are two reasons for this.

The first reason is that the diet works synergistically, as a whole. Nutrients must be balanced to work effectively. A very high dose of one nutrient may increase the need for another, thereby creating a deficiency that did not exist before. For example, vitamin A increases the need in the body for vitamin E; and vitamin E should be taken with selenium; very high doses of zinc may lead to iron deficiency. Nutrients do not work as well—or sometimes at all—in isolation. Picking and choosing foods will not be as effective as going on the whole diet.

The second reason is that there are several curious and largely unexplained anomalies in infertility that will be benefited by eating the diet as a whole. To name just one example: In studies of women who are prone to miscarriage, the husband often has low sperm counts. Though no study has ever shown that the woman's miscarriage occurs *because* of her husband's low sperm count, it would seem that, to be prudent, a diet to discourage miscarriage must also incorporate nutrients beneficial in raising the man's sperm count. Thus, try as much as is possible to follow the entire diet, rather than selecting and consuming the one or two nutrients that you think you most need.

How To Follow This Diet

Begin to incorporate the recipes into your daily diet. Different foods address different problems; and some foods are most effective taken in concert with other foods. In particular, you will be increasing your intake of yams, garlic, tofu and black soybeans, kelp, whole grains, cruciferous vegetables, alfalfa and leafy greens, pumpkin and sunflower seeds, almonds and walnuts, and wheat germ.

Do not attempt to pick and choose recipes based on "diagnoses" of your particular infertility problem. Instead, try to consume one food from each category each day. (You do not need to prepare a recipe from each section each day; although the recipes are listed under their principal ingredient, many of them contain more than one fertility-enhancing ingredient. In fact, as much as possible we have tried to include recipes that maximize your fertility with as little cooking as possible.) In any case, eat from all the food groups, rather than trying to diagnose your particular problem. Since exhaustive studies have not yet been undertaken, no one can be sure which foods do what. You will have better odds of conceiving by following the whole diet.

Vitamins

Although many of the nutrients discussed can be found in vitamin form, we recommend choosing the food equivalent rather than opting for the vitamin. One reason for this is that vitamin strategies alone can backfire: Too much of one vitamin (B6, for example) can create an imbalance of B vitamins; whereas elevating your B6 levels with whole foods does not present this problem.

Secondly, unpurified sources of nutrients can be harmful. Calcium from bone meal or dolomite, for example, has been found to be contaminated with lead, mercury, and arsenic; some herbal health pills have been discovered to contain lead.

Finally, too large a quantity of certain vitamins can be harmful, whereas an overabundance of a whole food is generally safe. Vitamins A and D, for example, are toxic if taken in doses only somewhat larger than the recommended daily allowance. To name another example, lecithin, a substance frequently found in vitamin supplements, in even slightly higher than normal doses, can cause brain abnormalities in rats. For all these reasons, we recommend eating foods to get your nutrients, rather than popping pills.

Diet as a Couple

Note that these recipes and food suggestions are for both women *and* men: Plan to go on the diet as a couple. Sperm count, sperm motility, and sperm morphology can all be affected by diet, as can female fertility conditions. Also, the added support of working together towards fertility will be motivating and encourage you to maintain the diet. And at least ten to fifteen percent of infertility is attributed to unknown causes. Since you can never be one hundred percent sure what is causing your particular fertility problem, do the diet together.

Diet for the Long Haul

Plan to stay on the diet for several months. Although sperm are produced daily, each sperm takes up to two and a half months to grow. And dietary changes, for both men and women, take time to yield benefits. In the same way that nutritional deficiencies *over long periods of time* may result in disease, nutritional corrections can only convey their benefits over time.

Whole Foods

Switch to a whole foods diet. All the research, not just on infertility but on everything from cataracts to cancer prevention, points to the value of a vegetarian, whole foods way of life. This means loading up on fruits, vegetables, and whole grains (such as brown rice, whole wheat flour, and oats), and dumping refined grains (such as white rice and white flour), processed foods and fatty meats.

Organic Produce

Use organic products as much as possible. The effects of consuming pesticides, chemicals, and growth hormones have not been sufficiently studied as to their impact on fertility, although a recent article in *The American Journal of Industrial Medicine* did draw the connection between pesticides and infertility.   And a Danish study published in *The Lancet* revealed that organic farmers who ate pesticide-free food were able to produce *double* the average quantity of sperm.

So play it safe: In the absence of conclusive scientific studies, strict adherence to a chemical-free, additive-free diet is certainly less risky.   Switch to organic fruits, vegetables, and milk products.   In particular, spinach, peanuts, raisins, strawberries, and peaches should be organic; together, these foods are estimated to contain over 25% of the average American's pesticide intake.   And anecdotal evidence has suggested that eating only organic bananas may be wise for fertility reasons.

Choose Your Oil Wisely

To cook your organic whole foods, we recommend sticking exclusively to olive oil and sesame oil.   Several years ago, a small town in rural China experienced a sudden, alarming drop in pregnancies, followed by an equally precipitous and inexplicable rise in pregnancy rate.   The phenomenon was investigated and it was learned that the only dietary change had been as a result of a shortage of the area's usual soybean oil; in its absence, cold-pressed cottonseed oil was substituted. As soon as the cold-pressed cottonseed oil was eliminated from their diet, fertility rose.

Today, cold-pressed cottonseed oil is used as birth control in some countries, because of its tendency to lead to decreased sperm production.

A related 1997 study in Nigeria examined the effects of feeding repeatedly thermoxidized palm oil (simulating a local Nigerian culinary practice) to rats.   Pregnancy rates were reduced by as much as fifty-five percent.   The Macrobiotic literature emphasizes the harmful effects of canola oil. Thus, the recipes in this book concentrate on olive and sesame oils. Note that other oils, cottonseed oil in particular, are found in many processed foods, including salad dressings.

No Smoking Section

Eating organic peaches will not be of much help if you are still smoking: Smokers have lower sperm counts, more abnormal sperm, and higher general infertility. Studies have also linked smoking to reduced levels of estrogen and poor cervical fluid. The bottom line is that more women who are smokers are infertile than nonsmokers.   Avoid smoking cigarettes completely.

Alcohol

Avoid alcohol. Although alcohol in moderation is now acknowledged for its possible health benefits at other times of life, it should be avoided completely during and while attempting pregnancy.

Even moderate drinking (one or two drinks a week) can elevate prolactin levels, inhibiting ovulation and leading to infertility. (For more information on the effects of elevated prolactin levels, see the chapter: Eating for Fertility: Specific Conditions.)

In addition, there was a *fifty* percent reduction in conception found in test animals given intoxicating doses of alcohol 24 hours prior to mating, according to a recent Science News article. Another recent study on alcohol showed that even one drink or fewer each week can reduce a couple's odds of conceiving that month by 40%. A 1998 study cited in *Fertility and Sterility* showed that women who consumed any alcohol had less than half the chance of becoming pregnant during a given cycle than abstainers. Their chances were even slimmer if they also drank more than 100 mg. of caffeine a day—the equivalent of about a cup of coffee.

Marijuana

Eliminate drugs. Marijuana is toxic to the developing egg and also hinders ovulation, according to a recent Science article.   Marijuana, and other hallucinogens, can elevate prolactin levels, causing infertility.   Alcohol and marijuana together cause drastic reductions in fertility in animals: In combination, offspring death rate ranged from 73% to 100%, according to information from the Research Institute on Alcoholism in New York.

Prescription And Non-Prescription Drugs

Avoid over-the-counter and prescription drugs as much as possible. Almost no studies have been done on the effects of these legal drugs on fertility.

In particular, headache and pain medication should be avoided, as it is thought that they might influence the quality of eggs produced. Headache and pain medication can also elevate prolactin levels, inhibiting ovulation.   Aspirin and nonsteroidal anti-inflammatory drugs (NSAIDS) such as Advil and Aleve should not be used since these may impede ovulation. Aspirin has also been linked to male infertility. Antihistamines and decongestants can dry up cervical fluid. Oral antibiotics can destroy the B vitamins and vitamin K, a deficiency of which can cause hemorrhaging in the placenta. Antidepressants can elevate prolactin levels, hindering ovulation.

Other drugs linked to male infertility include anabolic steroids, ulcer medication, UTI medication, anti-hypertensive drugs (specifically calcium channel blockers), epilepsy drugs, and certain antidepressants. And one side effect of certain high blood pressure medications is a tendency to ejaculate backward into the bladder (rather than forward out of the penis) effectively preventing fertilization. If you are currently taking any prescription drugs, be sure to discuss the issue with your doctor before discontinuing their use.

Caffeine

Eliminate caffeine, including coffee, chocolate, and soda. Anacin, Midol, and some cold remedies also contain caffeine.

Caffeine directly affects the nervous system, causing irritability, anxiety, and sleep disruption.   In addition to its miscarriage risks, high levels of caffeine have been implicated in delayed conception among otherwise fertile women. A 1997 study in the American Journal of Epidemiology observed that women with the highest levels of caffeine consumption had an increase in time leading to first pregnancy of eleven percent. (The effect was relatively stronger in women who also smoke.)   A 1998 study in *Fertility and Sterility* showed that women who consumed even small amounts of alcohol lowered their chances of pregnancy; their chances were even slimmer if they also drank more than 100 mg. of caffeine (about a cup of coffee) a day. In short, according to a recent study by the U.S. National Institute of Environmental Health Sciences, the more caffeine a woman consumes, the less likely she is to conceive. Women who drank one cup of coffee a day were half as likely to conceive as women who consumed no caffeine. (The good news is that the effects are short-term, so your past history of caffeine indulgence will not affect your future fertility.)

Although excess caffeine seems to impede fertility, tea, interestingly enough, seems to promote fertility. A recent study at Kaiser Permanente Medical Care Program of Northern California found that women who drank at least half a cup of tea each day were actually twice as likely to conceive as coffee and soda drinkers. Further studies must be done to confirm these findings, but researchers speculate that tea may contain chemicals that nurture the fertilized egg through the first weeks of life.   However, though it seems that tea may promote fertility, like all caffeinated beverages, it is implicated in miscarriage.   (Herbal tea eliminates the caffeine problem, but certain herbs are harmful to fertility; see the section "Herbs.")

Anecdotal evidence indicates that small amounts of caffeine, interestingly enough, may actually help sperm counts and sperm motility, but currently the research is inconclusive.

Aspartame

Avoid aspartame (NutraSweet and Equal).   Aspartame stimulates the pituitary gland to secrete prolactin, possibly causing elevated prolactin levels, which can prevent ovulation from occurring.   Diet foods including diet drink mixes, frozen desserts, gelatin, and soft drinks may contain aspartame.

Food Coloring

Food coloring should also be eliminated. The easiest way to do this, of course, is simply to cut processed foods from your diet. A 1997 study on the effect of food coloring on the reproductive abilities of mice showed a detrimental effect on testicular function and reproductive performance. Sperm count, sperm motility, and sperm morphology were all affected.

MSG

Monosodium glutamate (MSG) caused infertility in test animals, according to a study in *Neurobehavioral Toxicology*. It also caused brain damage in studies on infant animals, and has, for that reason, been removed from baby foods. Besides being found in Chinese and Japanese restaurants, MSG is found in Accent, many flavored potato chips, meat seasoning, and many packaged soups.

Vitamins

Women should avoid supplemental vitamin C.   Many women, trying to bolster their immune system before pregnancy or to avoid winter colds, begin taking megadoses of this vitamin. But vitamin C in large doses is an antihistamine, which can dry out cervical fluid. All the herbal literature points to the efficacy of supplemental vitamin C as a deterrent to pregnancy.   Just by eliminating their vitamin C intake, many women experiencing infertility problems have gone on to conceive. Note that natural vitamin C, in the form of citrus fruit for example, seems to be completely fine (maybe because you could not possibly approach that megadose quantity by eating oranges!)   The quantity of vitamin C in your multivitamin or prenatal vitamin should be insufficient to cause problems.

For men, though, vitamin C is necessary for fertility: It increases sperm motility, viability, and count. Vitamin C enhances the utilization of zinc, magnesium, copper, and potassium, which are vital to normal sperm functioning. In particular, vitamin C is helpful for men whose sperm clump together.

A 1996 study of fish at Ohio State University found that a high concentration of ascorbic acid in fish semen (reflecting dietary intake of vitamin C) played a key role in maintaining the genetic integrity of sperm cells, by preventing oxidative damage to sperm DNA. Thus, dietary ascorbate levels directly affect sperm quality and influenced male fertility positively in this vertebrate.

In a 1980 study, all of the wives of the men who received supplemental vitamin C became pregnant during the two month study. (None of the control group conceived.) Thus, vitamin C is indicated for men; it is only high doses of manufactured supplemental vitamin C that is harmful to women. Avoid it.

There is also some question in the herbal literature about consuming excess supplemental vitamin A and vitamin D. Again, although the amount in your multivitamin or prenatal vitamin is fine, curtail your intake of excess vitamins.

Ginger

Avoid ginger, which unfortunately is often *prescribed* for pregnant women suffering from nausea. Certainly do not consider consuming ginger if you have a history of miscarriage; it can actually cause miscarriage. Eliminate your consumption of ginger, ginger ale, and ginger beer. This topic is explored further in the chapter on miscarriage.

Quinine

Completely avoid quinine, the key ingredient in tonic water, quinine water, and bitter lemon. Quinine, used to cure malaria, has been linked to possible birth defects. (Note that tonic water should be distinguished from seltzer, which is not harmful.) The topic is explored further in the chapter on miscarriage.

Milk and More

The Macrobiotic literature on conception points to the following foods as harmful in the search for fertility: Meat, poultry, eggs, sugar (including honey and maple syrup; substitute brown rice syrup, barley malt, and molasses), chocolate, soda and diet soda, and seedless fruit (fruit with seeds is fine).   Cut down on these foods as much as possible. Milk and other dairy products are to be avoided.

Several studies show a negative correlation between milk consumption and fertility. According to a 1994 study done at Harvard Medical School and cited in the American Journal of Epidemiology, in countries where milk consumption is highest, women experience the sharpest age-related drop-off in fertility. Most adults lose the ability to easily digest lactose, a sugar in milk; this is apparently a beneficial loss, since lactose intolerance discourages high consumption of dairy products rich in galactose, and galactose is a sugar seemingly toxic to developing, unfertilized human eggs.   High rates of milk consumption thus correlate with waning fertility beginning in women just 20 years old; the correlation, and rate of fertility decline, grow with each successively older age studied. *Women with the highest concentrations of galactose are infertile.* Thus, avoid dairy as much as possible.

Another good reason to avoid dairy is its unbalanced ratio of calcium to magnesium, which inhibits the absorption of magnesium into the body. Magnesium deficiency can impede the working of the kidneys, causing fluid retention (and PMS). More importantly for fertility, magnesium deficiency has been linked to miscarriage: See the chapter on miscarriage for more information.

And Meat

Yet another good reason to avoid dairy, as well as meat, is dioxins. Dioxins are highly toxic, chlorinated byproducts of manufacturing processes (for example, combustion, incineration, and metal smelting.) Dioxins are created in the production of plastics, PVC, solvents, pesticides, wood preservatives, and disinfectants. When the waste containing these chlorines is burned, the dioxins are dispersed through the air, falling on the grass and plants, and are eventually consumed by animals.

Dairy and meat products are a major source of dioxins in humans. Dioxins do not dissolve readily in water, so plant and vegetable matter contains only small amounts of dioxins. But dioxins do dissolve readily in fat, so foods containing fat are heavily contaminated with dioxins. Studies indicate that between 80-90% of the average daily dioxin intake comes from eating milk and meat.

Dioxins affect the immune system, and are suspected of causing low sperm counts in men and endometriosis in women; numerous research studies have proven a link between dioxins and endometriosis in both monkeys and rodents. A 1979 study (Murray et al.) demonstrated decreased fertility in rats exposed to low levels of dioxins. Other studies have linked dioxin exposure to anovulation (failure to ovulate), decreased fertility, increased miscarriage rate, abnormal sperm morphology, and reduced male fertility. Whereas male subjects studied were not particularly sensitive to dioxins at low levels, female fertility was affected even at extremely low levels. Researchers at the Women's Environmental Health Network estimate that dioxins could affect as many as eight percent of unborn babies, and may affect their fertility in later life. It is also thought that dioxins could lead to a change in thyroid function, another link to endometriosis. Thus, for women in particular, dioxin exposure—and the eating of meat and dairy products—should be avoided.

If you decide to indulge in occasional meat meals regardless, be sure to strictly avoid the fat and fatty organs (kidneys, liver, brain) where most of the dangerous chemicals are concentrated. Stick to trimmed, lean meats. Poultry skin can also harbor undesired chemicals.

Finally, if you must have meat, order it well done. Undercooked meat can harbor a parasite that causes toxoplasmosis, a disease that is extremely dangerous to a developing fetus.

Cheese

A British study recommends avoiding all soft cheese. Because the processing does not involve pasteurization of the milk, the cheese can harbor the bacteria *Lysteria*, which can cause miscarriage.

Animal Fat

Another reason to avoid animal fat is the arachidonic acid it contains.   Arachidonic acid is a precursor of prostaglandin, which can impair the functioning of the corpus luteum, and thereby affect progesterone production in the luteal phase. Insufficient progesterone will not allow for a healthy endometrium.

Herbs

The herbal literature links the following to fertility difficulties: Basil, caraway seed, fenugreek, flax seed, fresh horseradish, licorice, marjoram, nutmeg, fresh rosemary, savory, tarragon, and watercress. Herbs such as burdock, catnip, celery seed, chamomile, cohosh, fennel, hyssop, juniper, mint, motherwort, mugwart, parsley, pennyroyal, saffron, sage, slippery elm, tansy, and thyme should be avoided, as they either promote menstruation or stimulate uterine contractions. A 1999 study at Loma Linda University School of Medicine in California linked the herbs St. John's wort, echinacea purpura, and ginkgo biloba to reduced sperm ability to penetrate the egg, as well as lowered sperm viability, and damaged sperm DNA. Avoid these herbs completely. Raspberry leaf tea, although touted by many as an anti-nausea drink for first trimester morning sickness, is also lauded as a way to induce uterine contractions and labor; therefore, it should be avoided.

Rhubarb and Peas

Rhubarb should be avoided, as it has been linked to infertility. Peas also have been linked to infertility; they seem to contain a natural contraceptive (m-xylohydroquinone) which interferes with estrogen and progesterone: In a study of rats fed 20% of their diet in peas, litter sizes were reduced, and 30% had no offspring.

Stress Reduction

Get some help in your efforts to relax. Stress levels almost certainly play some part in contributing to infertility. (Although it should be noted that stress only affects the woman's cycle when she is pre-ovulatory; the luteal phase, between ovulation and menstruation, is a constant length of time (which varies for individual women) and is unaffected by stress.) Therefore, though physical or emotional stress can temporarily delay ovulation, once ovulation finally occurs, stress will not impede the length of the luteal phase in that cycle.

Still, infertile couples who have learned to relax in support groups are statistically more likely to conceive than couples not in such groups. Dr. Alice Domar, psychologist and director of the Mind/Body Center for Women's Health at Beth Israel Deaconess Medical Center in Boston (affiliated with Harvard Medical School) and an associate of Dr. Herbert Benson, author of *The Relaxation Response*, did groundbreaking work in this area; her studies are still in progress, but her conclusions, that learning to relax, and talking about infertility within a supportive environment are helpful, seem incontrovertible.

While it is hard to relax under these trying circumstances, build some time into your schedule for it, and find some support for your attempts. Try meditation; enjoy a relaxation tape; find a support group. The appendix lists the addresses for several national infertility support groups.

Watch Your Weight

Before starting this diet, make certain that your weight is within the normal range for your height. If you are obese, the excess weight can lead to elevated estrogen levels, which impede the functioning of the corpus luteum and can prevent ovulation. Fat cells in women's bodies absorb and continually release estrogen. In obese women, the effect of constantly releasing estrogen suppresses the pituitary gland. At the onset of menstruation, because the pituitary gland is suppressed, there will not be as rapid and high an increase in follicle stimulating hormone necessary for ovulation to occur.

Obesity affects not only ovulation and response to fertility treatments, but also your ability to carry to term. Obese infertile women, *regardless of their infertility diagnosis*, who lose weight, become more fertile and become *significantly* more likely to carry to term. (In an Australian study in 1998, 18% miscarried, as opposed to 75% prior to the weight loss.) Thus, weight loss should be considered a basic first step for overweight women who are infertile.

Women with polycystic ovarian syndrome (PCO), should pay particular attention to their weight. PCO is the most common cause of anovulatory infertility and seems particularly vulnerable to the effects of excessive intake of calories. (Unfortunately, many women suffering from PCO find it particularly difficult to lose weight on a high-carbohydrate diet.) A 1996 study in England suggests that such women cut down on excess calories to maximize fertility. (For more information on PCO, see the section in "Specific Conditions".)

On the other hand, being underweight is also a potential pitfall: Studies that examined underweight dancers revealed that if you are more than ten to fifteen percent underweight for your size, you will stop ovulating. Too little body fat can cause scant fertile cervical fluid. The Macrobiotic literature also points to the importance of not being too thin. If you are not menstruating regularly, try gaining five pounds. If you are experiencing secondary infertility, try reattaining your previous (fertile) weight and build.

Crash Diets

Neither should you engage in crash diets. Crash dieting can cause a malfunction of the hypothalamus, resulting in reduced secretion of gonadotropin-releasing hormone. This can result in the disruption or cessation of follicle stimulating hormone, and the impossibility of a pregnancy.

(Nor should you diet strenuously after conception: Any harmful substances that you were exposed to prior to pregnancy are stored in your body's fat tissue. Dieting strenuously after conception could release those toxins into your baby's bloodstream.)

Furthermore, if you are seeking medical treatment for fertility, notify your doctor if you are suffering, or have suffered in the past, from an eating disorder. A Canadian study cited in *The American Journal of Obstetrics and Gynecology* showed that over 16% of infertile women had suffered from an eating disorder. Eating disorders can affect menstrual cycles, fertility, maternal weight gain, and fetal well being.

High Fat Diets

In addition to ensuring that you are a healthy weight, be certain to avoid excess dietary fat.   Impotence may be encouraged by a high-fat diet. In the same way that a high-fat diet contributes to hardening of the arteries, it may interfere with blood flow to the penis. Eliminating excess fat from the diet could solve your problem.

In addition, avoid fats created by deep-frying and trans-fats found in hydrogenated oils, including commercial cookies, breads, and margarines. Healthy sperm require long-chain fatty acids which may be displaced by trans-fatty acids. Thus, avoid trans-fats.

Protein

Cut down on your protein consumption. It is speculated that excess protein can impede fertility. Although no good studies on humans have been performed, a study cited in *The American Journal of Veterinary Medicine* showed that cattle that were fed excess protein showed a marked decrease in fertility rates and ova quality.

A 1998 study in Hong Kong showed a link between male subfertility and fish consumption, although it speculated that the increased level of mercury present was the likely culprit.

Although one study indicates that too strict a vegetarian diet can lead to irregular ovulation, we recommend sticking to a healthy, whole grain vegetarian diet that goes heavy on the fruits and vegetables, and avoids excess protein.

For women with recurrent miscarriage, however, inadequate protein is also a potential problem. The best middle ground seems to be that while you're attempting to conceive, eliminate excess protein; as soon as you have conceived, put that extra protein back into your diet.

Know When to Try

Your best chance of conception is if you are having intercourse in the few days immediately before ovulation. According to a recent study in *The New England Journal of Medicine*, among healthy women trying to conceive, nearly all pregnancies can be attributed to intercourse during the six-day period ending on the day of ovulation.

Ovulation *generally* (but not always) occurs halfway through your cycle. (In other words, if your period appears 28 days after the first day of your last period, ovulation would be happening at day number 14. In this case, you should have intercourse on days 9-13, particularly days 11-13.) However, not all women have 28 day cycles, and not all ovulate exactly at the mid-point of their cycle. Ovulation can occur as early as day eight (eight days after the onset of menstruation, that is) or as late as day 22.

Here are two ways to identify exactly when you should engage in intercourse to maximize your chance of conception. One is by measuring your morning temperature each day. Take your temperature first thing in the day—before getting out of bed or engaging in any activity. (Be sure you have had at least three *consecutive* hours of sleep beforehand.) When your temperature rises more than two-tenths of a degree higher than it had been on all of the previous six days, it means that you have ovulated. At this point, it is usually too late to attempt conception. However, as long as your temperature remains low (that is, less than two-tenths of a degree higher than on the six previous days), you can keep trying for conception—*no matter where you think you are in your cycle.* Thus, temperature can be used to confirm ovulation in hindsight, but by the time you have conclusively determined ovulation (by the temperature rise) you are usually no longer fertile and conception is unlikely. Thus, this method is not helpful for identifying impending ovulation, (and that is the most fertile part of your cycle.) It will show you, however, if you are indeed ovulating; and if there are at least ten days between the temperature rise and the first day of your menstrual cycle, it will determine that your luteal phase is long enough for implantation to occur.

The second way, which will actually predict the onset of ovulation in enough time for you to do something about it, is the quality of your cervical fluid. You are most fertile when your cervical fluid changes from dry or sticky to a stretchy, egg-white consistency. (On days when you have no cervical fluid, you are not fertile and will not be able to conceive.) In fact, although sperm can survive for as many as five days in fertile quality cervical fluid, if this cervical fluid is absent (i.e., you are dry) sperm can not live for more than an hour or two— not long enough to allow conception.

To learn more about these two methods of pinpointing ovulation, I highly recommend *Taking Charge of Your Fertility* by Toni Weschler.

Ovulation Kits

Ovulation kits on the market can be helpful, but to maximize your chances, you need to have had intercourse *before* the kit registers ovulation.   (Attempting intercourse within 24 hours of a positive reading can be successful.)

Also, ovulation kits test only for the luteinizing hormone surge that precedes ovulation, rather than ovulation itself. It is possible for women (particularly women over age 40) to have the luteinizing hormone surge, without actually proceeding to ovulate. If you are over 40 and experience exceptionally heavy menstrual flow, this may be due to an anovulatory cycle where an egg was not released. If your temperature did not rise, as discussed earlier, about two weeks before menstruation, the cycle is considered anovulatory. Also, the kits may register false luteinizing hormone surges which can occur several times before the real one; the danger here is that you will have intercourse too early for the sperm to survive until the real ovulation occurs.

Frequency of Intercourse

Couples where the man has low sperm count should engage in intercourse every other day during the fertile days; if the man has average counts, the couple should engage in intercourse every day to maximize chances of conception. (Do not wait more than two days between encounters, however; sperm motility tends to decrease with longer periods between ejaculations.) Traditional missionary position (man on top, woman underneath) will allow the greatest contact of sperm with cervical fluid, maximizing fertility. Finally, many reports indicate that the woman should lie down (for at least half an hour after the man ejaculates), before moving around, (for example, before going to the bathroom); a couple with marginal sperm count cannot afford to lose any sperm by leakage from the vagina. Obviously, do not douche after intercourse.

An extended period of sexual excitement will increase the amount of sperm present in the ejaculate, despite no increase in sperm production.

Be aware that large population studies of fertile volunteers have been found to have higher sperm counts in winter than in summer months, for no easily explicable reason.

Finally, engage in an active sex life! A six-month English study showed that in *fertile* couples, 16% of those who had intercourse less than once a week conceived within six months;

32% of those who had intercourse once a week; 46% of those who had intercourse twice a week; and 51% of those who had intercourse three times a week conceived within six months.

Avoid Excessive Exercise

According to a 1996 study in *The American Journal of Physiology*, when available energy is diverted to exercise, reproductive attempts are suspended in favor of physiological processes necessary for individual survival. Poorly controlled diabetes mellitus, eating disorders, cold exposure, and lactation can also account for infertility for this reason.

Too vigorous exercise also appears to lower sperm counts and negatively affects ovulation.

Unless You Produce Excess Estrogen

There is one situation in which you might want to consider engaging in vigorous exercise. According to current thinking, if you suffer from particularly heavy menstrual flow, it may well be because you are producing excess estrogen. If your infertility is linked to a production of excess estrogen, consider exercise as a possible remedy. A lifestyle of vigorous exercise will indirectly lower the production of excess estrogen.

Avoid the Dentist

Nitrous oxide can dramatically affect your ability to conceive, as well as your ability to sustain a pregnancy. Nitrous oxide is used in hospitals, veterinary clinics, and dental offices. Exposure is highest in dental offices, because masks are generally not placed on patients' mouths. (In other words, if you work in a dental office as a dentist, dental assistant, or dental hygienist, your fertility can be greatly compromised if your office uses nitrous oxide.) One study found that women experienced a 60% drop in conception rates after exposure to just five hours of nitrous oxide; 50% of the pregnant women in the study miscarried.

Avoid Vaginal Lubricants

According to a 1996 study, commercial vaginal lubricants inhibited sperm motility by 60-100% after sixty minutes of incubation; sperm viability was also detrimentally affected. Petroleum jelly, plain glycerin, *even saliva* can act as a spermicide and kill sperm. Thus, the use of vaginal lubricants during intercourse is definitely not recommended. In cases where a lubricant is required, the study suggests canola oil, which had no detrimental effects on motility or viability of sperm. We would recommend, instead, the use of egg whites (unless you have an allergy to eggs) since studies have shown that egg whites actually encourage sperm movement and are compatible with sperm viability.

Soaps and Shampoos

Switch to soap and shampoo made from all-natural ingredients. Many commercial soaps and shampoos contain alkyl-phynol ethoxylades, an estrogenic chemical thought to affect sperm count and quality. More studies need to be done to confirm this link, but in the meantime, buy all-natural soaps and shampoos from a health food store.

Plastic Wrap

Some plastic wraps contain endocrine disrupters which interfere with the body's hormones, leading to reproductive effects including low sperm count.   The dangerous plastic wraps are those that are composed of PVC and contain the plasticizer DEHA (di-(2-ethylhexyl)-adipate), the component that adds clinginess to the wrap.

Studies suggest that the DEHA plasticizer leaches onto food on contact.   In 1999, Consumers Union tested generic PVC cling wraps used to package supermarket deli cheese, finding that high levels of DEHA had migrated onto the cheese.

Polyethylene-based Handi-Wrap and Glad Wrap are apparently considered the best choices for cling wrap, as neither contain PVC.

Never use *any* plastic wrap in a microwave; Studies have conclusively proven the leaching of plastic into food in microwave use.

Although studies have not yet been conducted on PVC products other than cling wrap, couples worried about effects of PVC on fertility might choose to avoid all PVC plastics that come into contact with foods, including PVC containers.

Etc.

Read the suggestions in the miscarriage chapter. Once you have successfully conceived, you want to ensure that you carry the pregnancy to term without problem.

Finally try the suggestions in the appendix. Though these are anecdotal, rather than scientifically studied, they have worked for people.

Eating for Fertility: Specific Conditions

So your doctor has diagnosed your infertility problem. Are there specific nutritional suggestions that could be adopted by someone diagnosed with your particular infertility malady? Certainly. Should you follow those specific dietary recommendations? Not necessarily.

First of all, keep in mind that much infertility is still of unknown cause, or of more than one cause. Just because you suspect one malady does not mean that there is not more than one thing at play. By going on the diet as a whole, then, you will maximize your chances of dealing with infertility in general—whether or not you have been completely diagnosed.

Remember, too, that nutrients must be balanced to work effectively, and that this diet is designed to work synergistically. High doses of one nutrient, for example, may increase the need for another, causing a deficiency that did not formerly exist. Nutrients work best in combination with other nutrients, rather than in isolation. Picking and choosing nutrients is *not* the most effective way to enhance your fertility.

That being said, we have still chosen to include a section in this book arranged by specific condition. Primarily we have done so to encourage you to become as familiar with your body's specific nutritional needs as possible. Too, there might be foods on the diet that you dislike; if they are specific to your malady, you might be more prone to eat them. But we encourage you to use this information for education, and to *go on the diet as a whole*. That is still the best way to enhance your fertility.

Candida Albicans

Candida albicans, a naturally-occurring fungus, is the cause of vaginal yeast infections. Candida contributes to infertility by housing antibodies that affect the ovary, and by causing hormone imbalance and endometriosis.

Garlic is particularly effective against candida. Candida sufferers should also consume yogurt; soy, whole grains, walnuts, and wheat germ (for their pyridoxine, or vitamin B6, content); cruciferous vegetables (for the vitamin C and A); alfalfa (for the vitamin A and magnesium); and seeds and wheat germ (for the zinc). Avoiding yeast, sweets, and processed foods may also help.

Cervical Fluid

If the woman's cervical fluid is too acidic, sperm will not be able to survive, preventing conception. Among the old wives' tales discussing cervical fluid, cough syrup (ingested orally) is touted as a way to alkalinize the fluid; this method has never been proven.

What has been proven, however, is that antihistamines and decongestants can dry up cervical fluid, as can supplemental vitamin C. Avoid ingesting these substances if cervical fluid is a problem.

Endometriosis

If you suffer from terrible premenstrual syndrome, lower back pain, abnormal bleeding, depression, painful sex, and heavy periods, suspect endometriosis. An estimated five million American women suffer from endometriosis (including an estimated 30% of all infertile women.) If you have more than one symptom of endometriosis, consult your doctor.

Women with endometriosis should be particularly vigilant about increasing their consumption of kelp and wheat germ. Endometriosis has been linked to thyroid dysfunction and kelp is particularly good for thyroid problems. The vitamin E in wheat germ improves the healing of scar tissue caused by internal endometrial bleeding.

Women who suspect endometriosis should also cut down on their yeast consumption, as yeast overgrowth has been recently implicated in endometriosis. Correspondingly, since yeast thrives on sugar, strictly avoid sugar, as well as artificial sweeteners and dairy, though yogurt can be helpful for this problem.

In general, women with endometriosis should stick to a high-fiber, vegetarian based diet. Particularly, the elimination of fats from animal sources such as meat and dairy products is beneficial. Women with endometriosis should also particularly avoid caffeine and salt and should indulge in antioxidants such as sweet potatoes and yams, apricots, cantaloupes, carrots, spinach, and broccoli; as well as whole grains and beans for necessary B vitamins, and citrus fruits for bioflavonoids and natural vitamin C.

Endometrium

To ensure a healthy uterine lining, your diet must be adequate in vitamin A. Because vitamin E enhances the effect of vitamin A, and because selenium works synergistically with vitamin E, all of these nutrients should be consumed.

Eat more cruciferous vegetables, nuts, cantaloupe, asparagus, yams, spinach, and tomatoes (for vitamin A): whole grains, nuts, seeds, alfalfa, kelp, and wheat germ (for vitamin E); and garlic, whole grains, nuts, and wheat germ (for selenium).

Bioflavonoids also promote a healthy uterine lining. Eat more cruciferous vegetables, citrus fruit, and citrus fruit rinds (the latter are particularly tasty in baking.)

Estrogen/Progesterone Balance

If estrogen and progesterone levels are not balanced, it will be difficult to conceive. If estrogen levels are not elevated in the first part of the cycle, ovulation will not occur. If progesterone levels are not elevated in the second part of the cycle, a viable endometrium will not form.

Too much estrogen (which can manifest as particularly heavy menstrual flow) can sometimes be regulated by a vigorous program of exercise. Obesity can also cause elevated estrogen levels, so try to make sure that your weight is within the normal range. The dietary fiber in B6 vitamin-rich foods (tofu, kelp, whole grains, walnuts, and wheat germ) can also reduce estrogen levels.

Insufficient estrogen can be counteracted by increasing your consumption of para-aminobenzoic acid (PABA), which stimulates the pituitary gland into increasing estrogen production. Consuming wheat germ will satisfy your need for this nutrient.

Insufficient progesterone levels can be aided by increasing your consumption of foods rich in vitamin B6: tofu, kelp, whole grains, walnuts, and wheat germ. These foods can also reduce prolactin levels (which if present can be harmful to ovulation.)

Progesterone production in the luteal phase can also be affected if prostaglandin impairs the functioning of the corpus luteum. Avoid arachidonic acid, a precursor of prostaglandin, found in animal fat.

Finally, yams eaten in the pre-ovulatory part of the cycle are beneficial for women whose short luteal phase leads to insufficient progesterone production.

Hypothyroidism

Hypothyroidism is an underproduction of hormones by the thyroid gland, characterized by lowered cellular metabolism, including low basal body temperature and unexplained weight gain. Other symptoms can include accumulation of fluid under the eye, sensitivity to cold, aching muscles, decreased appetite (but concurrent weight gain), fatigue, constipation, dry skin and hair, insomnia, and tingling in the hands and feet. Reproductive symptoms include unusually long cycles and extended periods of heavy cervical fluid.

Hypothyroidism is perhaps one of the most common, yet easily overlooked causes of infertility. Hypothyroidism can throw the endocrine system off balance, causing elevated prolactin levels, which prevent ovulation. Thyroid secretion is essential not only for egg fertilization and development, but also for sperm production. Thyroid deficiency can now be identified by a thyroid stimulating hormone test, so see your doctor if you suspect thyroid deficiency.

Kelp, a sea vegetable, may help hypothyroidism, because of its high iodine content. Many people ingest enough iodine in their diet through the consumption of iodized salt. However, if you avoid processed foods and do not oversalt your foods; or if you are accustomed to using sea salt or kosher salt, neither of which contain added iodine, then kelp can fulfill this need. In addition, kelp may be better retained in the body, and is less likely to be readily excreted than salt.

If you have received a medical diagnosis of hypothyroidism, keep in mind that you should limit or avoid foods that inhibit the absorption of iodine in your system. These foods to avoid include peanuts, pine nuts, cabbage, mustard, and turnips.

Almonds and wheat germ are also helpful against hypothyroidism, as they contain dietary sources of vitamin B2 (riboflavin), a deficiency of which is linked to hypothyroidism. Avoid dried fruit, processed potatoes (dried, fried, or frozen), shrimp, and wine: The sulfites in these foods can destroy riboflavin, which can lead to a deficiency.

Luteal Phase Defects

A short luteal phase generally means that the corpus luteum does not produce sufficient progesterone, causing the onset of menstruation. Eating yams during the pre-ovulatory part of the cycle can correct a short luteal phase.

Insufficient progesterone levels can be aided by increasing your consumption of foods rich in Vitamin B6: tofu, kelp, whole grains, walnuts, and wheat germ.

Progesterone production in the luteal phase can also be affected if prostaglandin impairs the functioning of the corpus luteum. Avoid arachidonic acid, a precursor of prostaglandin, found in animal fat.

Miscarriage

Information on dietary approaches to preventing miscarriage is found in the chapter, "Preventing Miscarriage" on page 75.

Ovulation

Without ovulation, conception obviously can not occur.

Ovulation can be negatively affected by marijuana, aspartame, dioxins (in meat and dairy), and too strenuous exercise. As much as 25% of irregular ovulation can be attributed to elevated prolactin levels. See the section, "Prolactin."

Obesity can also suppress the pituitary gland, resulting in insufficient follicle stimulating hormone for ovulation to occur.

Consuming yams during the pre-ovulatory part of the cycle can sometimes stimulate ovulation: Yams act like the drug Clomid.

A deficiency of vitamin B6 (pyridoxine) can also elevate your prolactin level, which can suppress ovulation. Eat more soy, wheat germ, whole grains, and walnuts.

Polycystic Ovary Syndrome (PCO)

In PCO (also called Stein-Leventhal Syndrome) the body produces increased male hormones (androgens) which are converted into estrogen. In an obese woman, estrogen is also stored in the fat cells. Because estrogen is normally made from the developing follicles, the brain's hypothalamus, confused by the constant level of estrogen, assumes that it is due to a developing egg inside the follicle. Therefore, the hypothalamus tells the pituitary gland to stop or slow down the release of follicle stimulating hormone. Thus, the follicles don't mature and burst, and ovulation never occurs. Instead, the follicles turn into small cysts on the ovaries.

There have been very few good nutritional studies done on PCO, and the only nutritional recommendation currently given is that PCO sufferers should shed their excess weight. We have two suggestions: One is that you follow the general guidelines for anovulation. Consume yams, and elevate your levels of vitamin B6 (eat more soy, wheat germ, whole grains, and walnuts).

The second suggestion is, since PCO can often be characterized by elevated prolactin levels (the result of the constant estrogen levels associated with PCO) try following the dietary guidelines for elevated prolactin levels: Eliminate alcohol, marijuana, aspartame, dioxins in meat and dairy, too much protein, and too strenuous exercise.

Elevated Prolactin Levels

Normally, prolactin is released by the pituitary gland after pregnancy, to allow breastfeeding. It directly stimulates the breasts to produce milk and inhibits the release of follicle stimulating hormone and luteinizing hormone, thus preventing ovulation.

In women who are not post partum, elevated prolactin levels can be caused by a prolactin-microadenoma, a small, benign tumor in the pituitary gland. Other things that can raise prolactin levels include alcohol (even as little as one glass of wine a week); large consumption of protein; antidepressant medication; headache medicine; painkillers such as menstrual cramp medication; and hallucinogens such as marijuana. Aspartame, found in NutraSweet and Equal, can also raise prolactin levels. The high, constant level of prolactin hormone, if inappropriately present, in non-breastfeeding women, will cause a too-short luteal phase, inhibit ovulation, and thus cause infertility.   Polycystic Ovary Syndrome and Hypothyroidism can also be associated with elevated prolactin levels.

Vitamin B6 (in whole grains, soybeans, kelp, whole grains, walnuts and wheat germ) protects against elevated serum prolactin levels.

Prostaglandin

Prostaglandin can impair the functioning of the corpus luteum, adversely affecting progesterone production in the luteal phase.

Avoiding arachidonic acid, a precursor of prostaglandin, can correct this problem. Arachidonic acid is found in animal fat.

Sperm Count, Motility, and Morphology

Nutritional solutions are available for problems with sperm count, sperm morphology, sperm motility, and sperm clumping.

First of all, stick to olive and sesame oil; cottonseed oil, in particular, has been linked to decreased sperm production.

Other things that lower sperm count are smoking; food coloring; dioxins (from meat and dairy consumption); trans-fats (caused by deep frying and hydrogenated oils); and too vigorous exercise.

Vitamin C is beneficial, both to sperm count, motility, and morphology, as well as for men who have sperm clumping. Garlic, whole grains, and nuts are also helpful. (Nuts are particularly beneficial, both for their zinc content, and because they are one of very few foods containing arginine, which increases sperm count and motility.)

Preventing Miscarriage

Miscarriage is much more prevalent than is generally realized. Although the statistic bandied about of pregnancies resulting in miscarriage is 20-25%, that is the figure amongst women who are aware that they are pregnant. Studies conducted reveal that the true incidence of miscarriage is closer to *seventy* percent; the resulting slightly late, or slightly heavier than usual menstruation is actually very early miscarriage.

Many such miscarriages are not preventable, and are believed to be the result of unviable eggs. However, other miscarriages are preventable, and can be discouraged via nutritional improvements.

Most of the dietary guidelines for miscarriage prevention are the same as those for fertility promotion. Eat a whole foods, organic diet. Eliminate smoking, drugs, alcohol, and over-the-counter or prescription drugs as much as possible.

Increase your intake of yams, garlic, tofu and black soybeans, kelp, whole grains, cruciferous vegetables, alfalfa and leafy greens, pumpkin and sunflower seeds, almonds and walnuts, and wheat germ, and concentrate on olive or sesame oils.

Once you are pregnant, you can selectively add recipes and foods that contain lowfat milk, lowfat cheese, and occasional eggs and butter to your diet; these foods will bolster your protein and calcium content, and are not considered to be harmful once conception has occurred. However, it might be prudent to continue to restrict your dairy intake even after conception has occurred: Dairy has an unbalanced ratio of calcium to magnesium, which inhibits the absorption of magnesium into the body. Thus, it is possible that dairy can contribute towards a magnesium deficiency. (See the section in this chapter on "Alfalfa" for more information on why a magnesium deficiency may adversely affect pregnancy.)

Protein

Be sure to consume adequate protein, as protein deficiency has been linked to miscarriage. (For those on a vegetarian diet, this means combining foods that make proteins, such as beans and rice.) Keep in mind that fish, including easily prepared canned tuna and sardines, are good sources of protein if you are trying to cut back on dairy and meat.

Soy and Yams

If you are at risk of miscarriage, eat soy and yams, but *not* to tremendous excess. Particularly low estrogen levels created by excessive soy consumption cause a greater than 50% miscarriage rate in pregnant baboons, primates whose hormones are much like humans. Under 60 grams of soy protein per day is considered to be an acceptable dose; since ½ cup of tofu contains only eight (for regular tofu) or 15 (for firm tofu) grams of soy protein, it is unlikely (in fact, difficult) to overdose. (Moreover, in a recent study on rats, the genistein found in soy actually yielded a 50% reduction in breast cancer

in offspring—another good reason to indulge!)   There have
been no medical studies on the effects of overconsuming yams,
but since they are also phytoestrogens, they may exhibit the
same effect as soy. Therefore, eat yams, but not to excess.

Alfalfa

Pay particular attention to your intake of alfalfa which is
high in magnesium. A recent study in England showed a link
between magnesium deficiency and miscarriage rates. Because
magnesium is lost in the processing of many foods, the study
claimed that the magnesium content in the diets of North
American and English women is too low to support a healthy
pregnancy.

(This is the only hint in the medical literature as to why it
might be prudent to continue to restrict your dairy intake even
after conception has occurred: Dairy has an unbalanced ratio of
calcium to magnesium, which inhibits the absorption of
magnesium into the body. Thus, it is possible that dairy can
contribute towards a magnesium deficiency.)

Seeds and Wheat Germ

Zinc deficiencies have also been linked to increased risk of miscarriage, according to a recent Swedish study. Particularly if you also suffer from steatorrhea, inflammatory bowel disease, diabetes with insufficient metabolic control, alcoholism, or anything requiring treatment with diuretic drugs, up your zinc intake accordingly: Eat more pumpkin and sunflower seeds and wheat germ.

Thyroid

Low thyroid function has been implicated in miscarriage: Do not forget to eat kelp, almonds, and wheat germ.

Iron

Adequate iron guards against miscarriage and fetal malformation. Green leafy vegetables are a good source of non-animal iron. Molasses, chickpeas, dried apricots, and sardines are other good sources. However, large quantities of iron destroy Vitamin E, so supplemental iron should be avoided.

Vitamins

Deficiencies of vitamin E have also been linked to miscarriage. Among other things, vitamin E enhances the effect of vitamin A, necessary for a healthy endometrium. Although further studies need to be conducted, researchers have found that vitamin E is essential in the ability of pregnant animals to carry to term, and necessary for reproduction in general. Good food sources of vitamin E are whole grains, uncooked nuts, seeds, cabbage, spinach, asparagus, broccoli, alfalfa, rosehips, and seaweed. The single best natural source of vitamin E is wheat germ or wheat germ oil. If miscarriage is of particular concern, increase your intake of these vitamin E-rich foods.

Selenium works synergistically with vitamin E, and these foods should be eaten together. Note that although some amount of dietary iron is necessary to prevent miscarriage, supplemental iron destroys vitamin E, and should not be consumed in excess.

Also, completely avoid supplemental vitamin C. In addition to its role in drying out cervical lining, and thus possibly contributing to infertility, vitamin C in large doses is also implicated in miscarriage. Avoid except in your multivitamin.

Ginger

If you have had problems with miscarriage, *completely eliminate* ginger (also an ingredient in ginger beer, and some, though not all, ginger ale) from your diet. Ginger is referred to again and again in the herbal literature; it can be used to induce abortion. Evidence exists that women can bring on their menstrual cycle early, by as much as two or three days, simply by consuming ginger in quantity. But even small quantities of ginger can apparently be harmful. Taken by women who are trying to conceive, it may be an inadvertent cause of early miscarriage. Ironically, ginger is often prescribed for pregnant women who are experiencing morning sickness and while many women suffer no adverse effects from it, some significant number of women do. Avoid completely.

Quinine

Completely avoid quinine, the prime ingredient in tonic water, quinine water, and bitter lemon. (Note that tonic water is not the same as seltzer, which is harmless.) Although reliable studies have not been done, quinine is used in some countries as natural birth control; it has also been linked to birth defects.

Herbs

Herbs such as burdock, catnip, celery seed, chamomile, cohosh, fennel, hyssop, juniper, mint, motherwort, mugwart, parsley, pennyroyal, saffron, sage, slippery elm, tansy, and thyme should be avoided, as all either promote menstruation or stimulate uterine contractions. Raspberry leaf tea, although touted by many as an anti-nausea drink for first trimester morning sickness, is also lauded as a way to induce uterine contractions and labor; therefore, it should be avoided.

Cheese

Avoid consuming soft cheese British studies indicate that because the processing does not involve pasteurizing the milk, the cheese is at risk of harboring the bacteria *Lysteria* which can cause miscarriage.

Caffeine

A number of studies have linked miscarriage to caffeine intake. Apparently even a small amount of caffeine daily can increase your chances of miscarriage; certainly if taken in excess of two cups of coffee a day, caffeine can double your risk of miscarriage. To be absolutely sure, eliminate all caffeine from your diet: coffee, chocolate, tea, and soda. Surprisingly enough, *headache pills* often contain caffeine, so avoid these as well: a cold washcloth often is just as effective. Some cold remedies also contain caffeine.

Watch Your Weight

Be sure that your weight is within the normal range for your height. Obesity correlates directly to miscarriage. Obese infertile women, *regardless of their infertility diagnosis*, who lose weight become more fertile and *significantly* more likely to carry to term. In a 1998 study, 18% of women miscarried after weight loss, as opposed to 75% previously. Thus, weight loss should be considered a first step for overweight women at risk of miscarriage. Any weight within twelve pounds of your ideal weight is acceptable.

Birth Spacing

Close birth spacing has also been linked to increased risk of miscarriage. Researchers suspect that nutritional deficiencies resulting from attempts to conceive again too quickly result in mutagenic damage to both male and female germ cells, causing maldevelopment of the embryo. Therefore, be certain to give yourself adequate time between pregnancies.

Sperm Connection?

Women experiencing miscarriage typically have husbands with lower sperm counts and a higher degree of abnormal sperm, according to a recent Swedish study. So follow all the dietary guidelines designed to boost count and viability of sperm—even if you think your problem is miscarriage, rather than sperm.

Nail Polish Remover

Environmental pollutants have also been linked to miscarriage. *The British Journal of Industrial Medicine* includes a study showing a four-fold increase in spontaneous abortions in women working with chemical solvents, including acetone, also used in nail polish removers. Avoid! Miscarriage rates also increase after exposure to chemical solvents, according to a study by the University of California at Berkeley School of Public Health.

Dry Cleaning

Perchlorethylene and trichloroethylene, both of which are by-products of dry-cleaning, raised miscarriage rates 4.7 times and 3.1 times respectively. Paint thinners, paint strippers, and glycol ethers found in paints also raised the risks.

Nitrous Oxide

Nitrous oxide can dramatically affect your ability to sustain a pregnancy. Nitrous oxide is used in hospitals, veterinary clinics, and dental offices. Exposure is highest for workers in dental offices. One study found that exposure to just five hours of nitrous oxide resulted in miscarriages in half of the pregnant women in the study.

Night Lights

Try eliminating light (including digital clocks and street light) from your bedroom at night. One curious study showed a link between artificial night illumination and miscarriage.

Birth Defects

Finally, to prevent birth defects, increase your consumption of folic acid, docosahexaenoic acid (DHA) and iron. Deficiencies in folic acid can result in neural tube defects in newborns, including spina bifida and anencephaly. Folic acid deficiencies have also been implicated in miscarriage and threatened miscarriage, as well as premature birth. Leafy green vegetables are of particular importance in boosting folic acid levels, along with organic peanuts and beans.

Deficiencies in DHA have been linked to Attention Deficit Disorder and learning disabilities in children: Increase your intake of salmon, tuna, and sardines.

Iron nourishes the baby's red blood cells: Eat more chickpeas, beans, and lentils.

The Evidence Behind the Recipes

This section details the rationale behind the food suggestions, and provides recipes focusing on these "fertility-rich" foods.

Yams

Yams are full of antioxidants such as beta-carotene, which prevents heart disease, cancer, strokes, and cataracts.

Many cultures have linked yams to fertility promotion. Yams are promoted as fertility enhancers in the Ayurvedic literature. And studies on the native Yoruba tribe in Nigeria, which has one of the highest rates of twins in the world, suggest that their high rate of twins might be linked to their tremendous consumption of wild African yams.

Yams contain phytoestrogens, weak estrogens that inhibit the body's own estrogen. Acting much like the drug Clomid which is prescribed for women who are not ovulating, yams can apparently use this anti-estrogen effect to stimulate the ovaries to release an egg. (Like women given Clomid, Yoruba women have been shown to display high levels of follicle stimulating hormone in the first part of their cycle.)

Since it is apparently the high yam consumption that stimulates the release of more than one egg each month, scientists postulate that a daily diet of yams might increase one's chance of having fraternal twins.

Yams also are beneficial for women with short or inadequate luteal phases. For women whose corpus luteum does not make enough progesterone, thereby causing them to menstruate too soon, yams can regulate the hormones, contributing favorably to fertility.

Unfortunately, yams may also exhibit the same downsides as the drug Clomid: Although yams stimulate ovulation by increasing follicle stimulating hormone early in the cycle, it is possible that they can also counteract the effects of estrogen on the cervix (making the cervical fluid too sticky to allow sperm penetration) and the endometrium, (inhibiting the softening and receptivity of the uterine lining.) Therefore, like Clomid, yams should be consumed only during the first half of the cycle, not after ovulation.

Yams are also helpful in treating endometriosis and poor cervical fluid.

One cautionary note: *Excess* phytoestrogen is linked to a *decrease* in fertility in some animal studies, according to a recent article in *Gastroenterology*. Since the only applicable studies have been done on wild cheetahs, rather than humans, we recommend including yams in modest amounts. Do *not* consume yams in excess. (It would actually be difficult to consume yams in such quantity, unless you were on a yam diet where you consumed nothing else.)

Also note that yams are not the same as sweet potatoes. True yams are of the tuber family known as "Dioscorea" and bear only a superficial resemblance to American sweet potatoes. Nor is it known whether sweet potatoes convey the same fertility benefits as their look-alikes. Although some supermarkets mistakenly refer interchangeably to American sweet potatoes and yams, it is possible to find true Dioscorea yams. Ask in whole foods or health foods store for "true yams," or try markets specializing in Caribbean or African foods.

Garlic

Garlic, onions, scallions, leeks, radishes, and mustards, (in technicalese, "sulfur compounds") are all antioxidants. Raw garlic is a powerful antibiotic that fights parasites, viruses, and bacteria. It has cured encephalitis, heart disease, and stroke, and contains many anti-cancer compounds. It is good for colds, for boosting immunity, for lowering cholesterol and blood pressure, and as an antidepressant.

Garlic contains allicin, which destroys harmful bacteria in the body without interfering with the body's natural bacteria; thus its usefulness in fighting flu.

Garlic in particular seems to be effective against candida albicans, a naturally-occurring fungus which is the cause of vaginal yeast infections. Candida apparently contributes to infertility both by housing antibodies that affect the ovary and by causing hormone imbalance and endometriosis.

In addition to consuming garlic (yogurt is also helpful against candida), candida sufferers should avoid yeast, sweets, and most processed foods, and increase those foods rich in vitamin B6, vitamin C, vitamin A, magnesium, and zinc.

Garlic is also high in selenium, which raises sperm count and motility.

Tofu and Black Soybeans

Soy products (actually, the genistein found in soy) including tempeh, tofu, and soy milk, may not only prevent cancer and help inhibit tumor growth, but may also cause cancer cells to transform into normal cells. In pregnant lab animals, genistein led to a 50% reduction in breast cancer in the offspring.

In terms of fertility, soy products are high in vitamin B6, a deficiency of which causes all sorts of fertility problems, from estrogen-progesterone imbalance to elevated serum prolactin levels. (If B vitamins are insufficient, the liver can not inactivate estrogen, and the maintained high estrogen levels will reduce the necessary progesterone levels. And elevated serum prolactin can interfere with ovulation.) Vitamin B6 also helps against Candida Albicans.

Mixing circumin with the genistein in soy enhances its reproductive effects still more.   Circumin is the active ingredient in turmeric root.   Thus, combining turmeric with soy, as in many Indian curries, will boost soy's reproductive effects.

Tofu also contains calcium, which can compensate for a deficiency of vitamin D, known to cause infertility in animals.

Black soybeans are particularly singled out by the macrobiotic literature as effective fertility promoters: Wendy Esko, a macrobiotic counselor with the Kushi Institute in Beckett, Massachusetts, recommends both black soybeans and black soybean tea for fertility enhancement.

One cautionary note: Excess phytoestrogen, the weak estrogen contained in soybean protein, is linked to a *decrease* in fertility in some animal studies, according to a recent article in *Gastroenterology*.   Since the only applicable studies have been done on wild cheetahs, rather than humans, we recommend including soy products, but in modest amounts. Do *not* consume soy in excess.

Further, there is some question that blunting the estrogen effect too much may increase the risk of miscarriage. Although Chinese and Japanese women on diets quite high in soy do not have miscarriage problems as a result, low estrogen levels do create a greater than 50% miscarriage rate in pregnant baboons, primates whose hormones act much like humans. Thus, for both these reasons, do *not* consume soy in excess. Sixty grams per day is considered a safe dose. Since raw tofu contains only eight grams per half cup (for regular tofu) or fifteen grams per half cup (for firm tofu), it is unlikely that you would approach a dangerous dosage unless you were also supplementing with genistein tablets, which we do not recommend. Soy milk has much less genistein, and is not as useful as tofu for boosting these levels; soy sauce and soyburgers are even worse in terms of their genistein content.

Kelp

Hypothyroidism is an underproduction of hormones by the thyroid gland, characterized by lowered cellular metabolism, including low basal body temperature and unexplained weight gain. Other symptoms can include accumulation of fluid under the eye, sensitivity to cold, aching muscles, decreased appetite (but concurrent weight gain), fatigue, constipation, dry skin and hair, insomnia, and tingling in the hands and feet. Reproductive symptoms include unusually long cycles and extended periods of heavy cervical fluid.

Hypothyroidism is perhaps one of the most common, yet easily overlooked causes of infertility. Hypothyroidism can throw the endocrine system off balance, causing elevated prolactin levels, which prevent ovulation. Thyroid secretion is essential not only for egg fertilization and development, but also for sperm production.   Thyroid deficiency can now be identified by a thyroid stimulating hormone test, so see your doctor if you suspect thyroid deficiency.

Kelp, a sea vegetable, may help hypothyroidism, because of its high iodine content. Many people ingest enough iodine in their diet through the consumption of iodized salt. However, if you avoid processed foods and do not oversalt your foods; or if you are accustomed to using sea salt or kosher salt, neither of which contain added iodine, then kelp can fulfill this need. In addition, kelp may be better retained in the body, and is less likely to be readily excreted than salt.

If you have received a medical diagnosis of hypothyroidism, keep in mind that you should limit or avoid foods that inhibit the absorption of iodine in your system.

These foods to avoid include peanuts, pine nuts, cabbage, mustard, and turnips.

Kelp is also helpful for the treatment of endometriosis. Between ten and 20% of women are affected by endometriosis, though symptoms only manifest in some women. Endometriosis is suspected as the cause of infertility in 30% of all infertile women.

It is believed by some researchers that women with endometriosis may be suffering from a thyroid dysfunction. Of 120 women with endometriosis in one study, although thyroid tests had been normal, the incidence of thyroid antibodies was 20% higher than in the control group.

Kelp is also rich in the B-complex vitamins, vitamins D, E, and K, calcium, and magnesium, all of which enhance fertility. Kelp's Vitamin B6, in concert with its magnesium, is also synergistic prevention against edema, toxemia, and eclampsia. Kelp is considered a natural antiviral and antibacterial food, and has been shown to lower blood and cholesterol levels.

Whole Grains

Whole grain products, including whole wheat bread and brown rice, are high in vitamin B6, helping to maintain estrogen/progesterone balance and normal serum prolactin levels. (Elevated serum prolactin can interfere with ovulation.) Vitamin B6 also helps against candida albicans.

Because too much of a B vitamin taken alone can cause an imbalance, when doctors see a deficiency in one B vitamin, they generally prescribe a B-complex supplement. However, elevating your levels of B6 with whole foods does not present this problem.

Whole grains are also high in selenium. Populations living where there is selenium-rich soil have a higher birth rate than selenium-deprived areas, and there is believed to be a connection with sperm production. At least half of the selenium in the male body is found in the semen, and selenium has been shown to avert infertility in animals. A 1998 study in *The British Journal of Urology* showed that selenium supplementation in subfertile men improved sperm counts and motility, and thus the chance of successful conception: 56% showed a positive response to selenium treatment.

Whole grains also house vitamin E, linked to increased sperm count and helpful in endometriosis, as well as miscarriage prevention.   And of course, the effect of the vitamin E is enhanced by the concurrent consumption of selenium.

Finally, whole grains contain chromium, a deficiency of which, in animals, was accompanied by a decreased sperm count.

Cruciferous Vegetables

Indoles, specifically indole-3 carbinol, found in cruciferous vegetables including broccoli, brussel sprouts, cabbage, bok choy, collards, kale, and cauliflower, have been linked to the reduction of breast and other cancers. Broccoli, and in particular, broccoli sprouts, have been found to be packed with cancer-fighting sulforaphane.   Note that indoles can be deactivated by heat; thus, do not cook these vegetables to death.

For infertility, cruciferous vegetables are promising because of the high vitamin C count, particularly in broccoli, cauliflower, Chinese cabbage, kale, and mustard greens (as well as cantaloupe, berries, and citrus fruits.) Ascorbic acid in supplemental vitamin C *has* been linked to very early miscarriage, however, sperm motility, viability, and count have all improved. Vitamin C has also been shown to be particularly helpful for men whose sperm tend to clump together. Vitamin C in its natural form (that is, in foods) has *not* been linked to early miscarriage the way the vitamin supplements have. Vitamin C is also helpful against candida albicans.

In addition, the bioflavonoids in many cruciferous vegetables and citrus fruit rinds seem to promote a healthy uterine lining.

And the vitamin A that occurs in cruciferous vegetables, as well as in such foods as cantaloupe, asparagus, yams, spinach and tomatoes, may be linked to the production of healthy sperm cells, as well as helpful against candida. Note, though, that vitamin A increases the body's need for vitamin E (and therefore selenium) so do not forget to also eat your wheat germ, nuts, and seeds.

Also, it seems that a vitamin D deficiency (which in animals can reduce fertility by 75 percent) can be counteracted by sufficiently high doses of calcium. Broccoli and kale are particularly high in calcium.

Broccoli also houses selenium, helpful for sperm count and motility.

Alfalfa and Leafy Greens

Alfalfa is high in iron, magnesium and calcium, making it particularly useful in the treatment of endometriosis.

Its high magnesium content, in particular, is beneficial in preventing both candida and miscarriage.

A recent study in Wales and England showed that magnesium during pregnancy reduced miscarriage, and suggested that the diets of most North American and European women are too low in magnesium to support a healthy pregnancy. Magnesium is lost in the processing of many foods. Subsequent studies on the effects of magnesium on animal fertility seem to confirm this link. Note, too, that calcium and magnesium, both of which are housed in alfalfa, must be taken together to prevent magnesium deficiency.

Alfalfa is also high in vitamin E, which is essential for many facets of the reproductive process. It contains vitamins A, K, B, and D. It is high in protein and contains phosphorous, iron, potassium, chlorine, sodium, and silicon.

Leafy greens, particularly kale and mustard greens, are high in folic acid, vital for both fertility and the prevention of birth defects. Leafy greens are also particularly cited by the Macrobiotic literature as necessary for fertility.

Leafy greens are also high in vitamin K, a deficiency of which can cause hemorrhaging in the placenta.

Leafy greens are also a good non-animal source of iron, an adequate amount of which guards against miscarriage and fetal malformation.

Pumpkin and Sunflower Seeds

Seeds are particularly high in zinc, a deficiency of which is linked to low sperm count. Even a marginal zinc deficiency has caused sperm counts to drop precipitously; the highest concentrations of zinc in the body are found in the sperm and the prostate gland. Low sperm motility is also helped by zinc, as is potency and sexual desire. Zinc also affects female fertility, particularly in concert with vitamin B6.

Though studies on humans are scanty, several studies on animals have strengthened suspicions of a zinc deficiency-infertility connection. A Sudanese study linked zinc deficiency to infertility in cattle. A later French study cited a beneficial connection between zinc supplementation and increased fertility in human females. Zinc is also helpful against candida albicans.

Zinc deficiency is also implicated in miscarriage. According to a recent Swedish study, particularly if you also suffer from steatorrhea, inflammatory bowel disease, diabetes with insufficient metabolic control, alcoholism, or anything requiring treatment with diuretic drugs, you should increase your consumption of zinc.

Raw Almonds and Walnuts

Nuts, particularly almonds and walnuts, are loaded with vitamin E, necessary for overall fertility. Most reports indicate that the nutrients in nuts may be lessened with the cooking process; therefore, the recipes mostly call for the raw nuts as a garnish, rather than a cooked ingredient.

Nuts are also one of the few foods (chocolate is another) containing arginine. Arginine, a non-essential amino acid, has been discovered to markedly increase sperm count and motility.

Walnuts' high level of vitamin B6 protects against candida, estrogen/progesterone imbalance, as well as elevated serum prolactin levels, which can prevent ovulation.

Both the herbal and Ayurvedic communities cite raw almonds in particular as a fertility enhancer. Almonds do contain dietary sources of riboflavin, vitamin B2, a deficiency of which is linked to hypothyroidism.

Brazil nuts are high in selenium, which can aid in sperm production. However, because brazil nuts can be toxic if taken in large quantities, do not take more than *one* brazil nut each day.

Wheat Germ

Vitamin E has a dramatic effect on the reproductive organs; it increases male and female fertility and helps restore male potency. A vitamin E deficiency may be linked to low sperm count in men, and endometriosis in women. Researchers found that vitamin E is essential in the ability of pregnant animals to carry to term, and necessary for reproduction in general.

Studies have also linked vitamin E to sperm's impregnating ability: Vitamin E helps sperm attach better to the egg. Later on, vitamin E helps prevent against miscarriage. Finally, vitamin E improves the healing of scar tissue causes by internal endometrial bleeding. Vitamin E can correct menstrual rhythm and combined with other nutrients, may be a replacement for estrogen therapy. Good food sources of vitamin E are whole grains, uncooked nuts, seeds, cabbage, spinach, asparagus, broccoli, alfalfa, rosehips, and seaweed. The single best source of vitamin E is wheat germ or wheat germ oil.

Wheat germ is also high in selenium, which averts infertility in animals. A 1998 study in *The British Journal of Urology* showed that selenium supplementation in subfertile men improved sperm counts and motility, and thus the chance of successful conception.

Wheat germ is also high in vitamin B6, Pyridoxine, helping to maintain estrogen/progesterone balance and normal serum prolactin levels. (Elevated serum prolactin can interfere with ovulation.) It will also help with candida.

Wheat germ is a source of riboflavin, vitamin B2, a deficiency of which is linked to hypothyroidism.

Wheat germ is high in zinc, linked to increased sperm count and motility, and miscarriage prevention.

Finally, wheat germ contains para-aminobenzoic acid (PABA), which taken along with folic acid, has been shown to stimulate the pituitary gland and increase estrogen levels, and greatly improved the ability of women who have a history of infertility to conceive.

Questions

Q: I've been trying to get pregnant for eight months, but I haven't seen a doctor yet. Can this diet help me even though I don't know what the problem is?

A: We've included information on dietary changes that can benefit particular problems, but all of the nutritional suggestions are safe and beneficial for anyone struggling with fertility, whether you have been diagnosed with a particular problem or not.

Also, bear in mind that you may not *have* a problem—perhaps you have been inaccurate in pinpointing your ovulation—or you may not have a medically diagnosable problem: At least ten to fifteen percent of infertility is attributed to unknown causes. For all these reasons, the nutritional suggestions in this book may be beneficial.

Q: My doctor told us why we're infertile. Can't we just read the information that pertains to our problem and follow those recommendations, and not worry about the rest of the diet?

A: While we certainly can't prevent you from taking that approach, it's really not in your best interests. As we've pointed out, nutrients work synergistically, and must be balanced to work effectively. Picking and choosing foods is not as healthy, or as likely to succeed, as going on the diet as a whole. Furthermore, there are some curious anomalies in infertility that are benefited by approaching the diet as a whole. (For example, women who are prone to miscarry are more likely to have husbands with low sperm counts.) Thus, picking and choosing nutrients is not as effective as following the entire diet.

Q: We've been on the diet for a month, but still haven't conceived. Does that mean it's not working for us?

A: Maybe. But it's equally likely that you haven't given it enough time. For example, although sperm are produced daily, the production of individual sperm can take two and a half months. Dietary changes, for both men and women, take time to yield benefits. And in the same way that nutritional deficiencies may result in disease whenever inadequate nutrients are consumed over long periods of time, nutritional benefits can be expected only over time as well.

Q: I'm about 25 pounds overweight. Does that have anything to do with my infertility?

A: Although some women who are overweight find it possible to conceive, many others do not. In general, women who are overweight have elevated estrogen levels, which can prevent ovulation. In addition, obesity affects not only ovulation, but also ability to carry to term: Obese women who lose weight are significantly more likely to be able to carry to term.

Q: I conceived easily the first time, but now seem to have secondary infertility. Could my recent weight loss be at fault?

A: Yes; being underweight can prevent ovulation and cause insufficient cervical fluid. Try reattaining your previous (fertile) weight and build.

Q: Is there a best time of year to attempt conception?

A: Interestingly enough, sperm counts were found to be higher in winter months than summer months. So it's possible that couples with a sperm count problem could benefit from attempting conception in the winter. (On the other hand, more people seem to get sick in the winter, and many medicine cabinet cold drugs are detrimental to fertility, including aspirin, anti-inflammatory drugs, antihistamines, decongestants, vitamin C and oral antibiotics.)

Q: My husband and I are long-distance runners. Could that have something to do with our inability to conceive?

A: Vigorous exercise has been linked both to low sperm counts and inability to ovulate in some people. Try switching to less vigorous activity—yoga, walking, or swimming—and see what happens.

Q: My doctor says I produce too much estrogen. Any ideas?

A: Excess estrogen production (which can manifest as particularly heavy menstrual flow) can be counteracted by engaging in vigorous exercise. Try a heavy exercise program to see if you can lower those estrogen levels.

Elevated estrogen levels can also be caused by obesity, so make sure your weight is within the normal range for your height to maximize fertility.

Q: I have the opposite problem: I don't produce enough estrogen.

A: Para-aminobenzoic acid (PABA) has been shown to stimulate the pituitary gland and increase estrogen levels. Get your daily dose by eating wheat germ.

Q: Apparently I don't produce enough progesterone. Are there nutritional remedies for this problem?

A: B vitamins allow the liver to inactivate estrogen, thus allowing for the production of progesterone. Vitamin B6 in particular can elevate progesterone levels. Try increasing your consumption of tofu, kelp, whole grains, walnuts, and wheat germ.

Progesterone production in the luteal phase can also be affected if prostaglandin impairs the functioning of the corpus luteum. Avoid arachidonic acid, a precursor of prostaglandin, found in animal fat.

Finally, yams, taken in the first half of the cycle (pre-ovulation) are beneficial for women with short luteal phases whose corpus luteum does not make enough progesterone, thereby causing the too-early onset of menstruation.

Q: I suffer from endometriosis. Are there dietary changes that will correct it?

A: Although diet may not be able to alleviate endometriosis, nutritional changes can often enhance fertility in spite of endometriosis. Because endometriosis has been linked to thyroid dysfunction, make certain that you are consuming kelp, which is particularly helpful for thyroid problems. Furthermore, women with endometriosis should be vigilant about consuming wheat germ: The vitamin E in wheat germ improves the healing of scar tissue caused by internal endometrial bleeding. Finally, cut down on yeast, sugar, artificial sweeteners, salt, caffeine, and dairy, and stick to a high-fiber, vegetarian diet, eliminating all dietary fat from animal products.

Q: What can I do nutritionally for candida albicans?

A: Candida albicans, a naturally-occurring fungus which causes vaginal yeast infections, apparently contributes to infertility by housing antibodies that affect the ovary and by causing hormone imbalance and endometriosis.

Dietary approaches to candida include garlic; yogurt; soy, wheat germ, whole grains, and walnuts for vitamin B6; cruciferous vegetables for vitamin C; and cruciferous vegetables and alfalfa for vitamin A. Avoid yeast, sweets, and processed foods.

Q: My doctor says my problem is elevated prolactin levels that are preventing ovulation. Is there anything I can do for that?

A: In a normal, post-partum woman, prolactin is released to allow breastfeeding. It directly stimulates the breasts to produce milk, and inhibits the release of follicle stimulating and luteinizing hormones, thus preventing ovulation. In women who are not post-partum, elevated prolactin levels can be caused by a prolactin microadenoma, a small benign tumor of the pituitary gland. It can also be the result of marijuana, alcohol, pain medication, or antidepressants. Interestingly, aspartame can also cause elevated prolactin levels. The high constant level of prolactin will cause a too-short luteal phase, inhibiting ovulation and thus impeding fertility.

Vitamin B6, in whole grains, soybeans, kelp, walnuts, and wheat germ, protect against elevated prolactin levels.

Q: I've had three miscarriages. Can this diet really help with miscarriage?

A: Miscarriage has been linked to deficiencies in magnesium, zinc, iron, vitamin E, and vitamin A. Eating a diet rich in these nutrients will certainly enhance your ability to carry to term. Miscarriage is also linked to the consumption of various foods—ginger; vitamin C; quinine in quinine water, tonic water, and bitter lemon; unpasteurized soft cheese; certain herbs; and caffeine, including that in headache pills. Finally, there are several environmental factors implicated in miscarriage. Read the chapter "Preventing Miscarriage" for more details.

Q: I've been diagnosed with a problem with my endometrium. Can nutrition affect that?

A: To ensure a healthy endometrium, or uterine lining, your diet must be adequate in vitamin A. In addition, vitamin E enhances the effect of vitamin A, and selenium works synergistically with vitamin E, so all these nutrients should be consumed. In terms of food, this means cruciferous vegetables, nuts, cantaloupe, asparagus, yams, spinach, and tomatoes for vitamin A; whole grains, nuts, seeds, alfalfa, kelp, and wheat germ for the vitamin E; and garlic, whole grains, nuts, and wheat germ for selenium.

Bioflavonoids also promote a healthy uterine lining: Dietary sources of bioflavonoids include cruciferous vegetables and citrus fruit rinds.

Q: I have hypothyroidism. I eat kelp; is there anything else I can do?

A: Two things. One is to limit or avoid foods that inhibit the absorption of iodine in your system. Foods to avoid include peanuts, pine nuts, mustard, cabbage, and turnips.

The second is to increase your dietary intake of riboflavin, vitamin B2, a deficiency of which is linked to hypothyroidism. You can get dietary riboflavin in wheat germ and almonds. Simultaneously, avoid dried fruit, processed potatoes, shrimp, and wine; the sulfites in these foods destroy riboflavin.

Q: Can nutrition help with low sperm count?

A: Nutrition can help with low sperm count, as well as sperm morphology, sperm motility, and clumping of sperm. First of all, stick to olive and sesame oil; cottonseed oil, in particular, has been linked to decreased sperm production. Other things that lower sperm count are smoking, food coloring, dioxins (from meat and dairy), trans-fats caused by deep frying and hydrogenated oils, and vigorous exercise.

Vitamin C is beneficial, both to sperm count, motility, and morphology, as well as for men who have sperm clumping. Garlic and whole grains, are also beneficial. Nuts are helpful, both for their zinc content and because they are one of the few foods containing arginine, which increases sperm count and motility.

Women who miscarry typically have partners with low sperm counts, and a higher degree of abnormal sperm, according to a recent Swedish study. So even though a causal link has not yet been established, boosting healthy sperm levels may also reduce miscarriage odds.

Q: I'm not certain whether I'm ovulating. How can I tell?

A: Read the section "Know when to try" in "Eating for Fertility." You can not only determine if you are ovulating, but calculate the exact time of ovulation, through a combination of temperature and cervical fluid reading.

Q: Are ovulation kits accurate?

A: Yes and no. They are generally accurate in that they pinpoint ovulation for most women. To maximize your chance of conception, however, you need to have had intercourse before the kit registers ovulation, although attempting intercourse within 24 hours can be successful.

In addition, they register the luteinizing hormone surge that precedes ovulation, but it is possible for women to experience the LH surge without going on to ovulate, particularly for women over 40. Furthermore, there can be more than one LH surge; if the kit registers an early (false) surge, you might end up having intercourse too early for the sperm to survive until the true ovulation occurs.

Q: I don't ovulate. How can I change my diet to correct this problem?

A: First of all, try eliminating any of the following that you indulge in: marijuana, aspartame, dioxins (in meat and dairy), and vigorous exercise.

Second, be sure that you're not overweight: Obesity can suppress the pituitary gland, resulting in insufficient follicle stimulating hormone. Try eating yams during the pre-ovulatory part of your cycle; they can imitate the drug Clomid and cause ovulation.

And finally, eat more soy, wheat germ, kelp, whole grains, and walnuts, for their pyridoxine (vitamin B6) content, a deficiency of which can elevate your prolactin levels, suppressing ovulation.

Q: Is there anything to be done about a short luteal phase?

A: Try eating yams during the pre-ovulatory phase.

Q: I've been diagnosed with hostile cervical fluid. Is there anything I can do for it? Someone suggested cough syrup, but that hasn't worked for me.

A: Eliminate   antihistamines,   decongestants,   and supplemental vitamin C if you have been taking them. All of these can dry up cervical fluid.

Menu Planning

Remember, in formulating your menus, try to include something from each food group each day. This does not always mean that you will need to prepare one recipe from each section; many of the recipes contain more than one fertility food. Remember to look at the recipes themselves: Yam and Apple Casserole, for example, also supplies the day's requirement of sunflower seeds and almonds.

Remember that women attempting to conceive should avoid recipes containing dairy. Women who have conceived, but are following the diet to avoid miscarriage, can reintroduce recipes with low fat dairy.

I find it easiest to plan the main meal of the day first. Once I have crossed off a few food groups that will become part of our dinner, it is easy to go back and plug the missing food groups into lunch. As for breakfast, we like to alternate between sweet, traditional breakfast fare (whole grain pancakes, muffins, cereals) and savory grains with sauces, and porridges. And of course it is easy to pick up the balance of the foods in a mid-afternoon snack, which can range from raw seeds and nuts to yam fritters or soybean nibbles.

Here is a handy planner you can adapt to use in tracking your diet. Simply check off the appropriate categories to ensure that everything is covered. We have filled out a sample day as an example. Notice how some dishes cover several categories at once. You might want to copy the blank plan to use in your daily menu planning.

Example menu:

Breakfast:	Wheat Germ Cereal with Yogurt
Lunch:	Ratatouille, served over brown rice
Snack:	Sunflower seeds
Dinner:	Indonesian Tofu; Green Yam Salad

Food Categories Covered:

Category:	**Dish:**
Yams:	Green Yam Salad
Garlic:	Indonesian Tofu
Tofu & Black Soybeans:	Indonesian Tofu
Kelp:	Ratatouille
Whole Grains:	Wheat Germ Cereal (oats); Ratatouille served over brown rice
Cruciferous Vegetables:	Indonesian Tofu
Alfalfa & Leafy Greens:	Green Yam Salad
Pumpkin & Sunflower Seeds:	Sunflower Seed Snack
Almonds and Walnuts:	Wheat Germ Cereal
Wheat Germ:	Wheat Germ Cereal

Your menu:
> Breakfast:
> Lunch:
> Snack:
> Dinner:

Food Categories Covered:
> **Category:**   **Dish:**
> Yams:
> Garlic:
> Tofu & Black Soybeans:
> Kelp:
> Whole Grains:
> Cruciferous Vegetables:
> Alfalfa & Leafy Greens:
> Pumpkin & Sunflower Seeds:
> Almonds and Walnuts:
> Wheat Germ:

Sample Menus

The dishes below that appear in italics are included in this cookbook. This menu plan also includes a few dishes whose recipes are not included, such as mixed seeds for snackfood and simple steamed greens. Remember that you can use these sample menus as a basis without rigid adherence to them: If you would like your wheat germ sprinkled over your salad instead of your granola, go right ahead. Just make sure you are eating from each of the food groups as much as possible.

And remember that women who have not yet conceived should eliminate all recipes with dairy—or simply eliminate the dairy from the recipes.

Breakfast: *Granola* (whole grains, almonds, seeds) sprinkled with wheat germ

Lunch: Steamed Greens and Cauliflower with *Tofu Dressing* (leafy greens, cruciferous vegetables, tofu) in pita pocket

Dinner: *Curried Barley Soup* (kelp, whole grains, garlic); *Cheesy Yams* (yams)

Breakfast: *Yam Muffins* (whole grains, yams)

Lunch: Mug of *Tofu Chowder*; Alfalfa and Leafy Greens with *Broccoli Pesto*, and garnished with seeds, nuts and wheat germ

Dinner: *Walnut Risotto with Garlic* (walnuts, whole grains, garlic)

Breakfast: Leftover *Tofu Chowder* over brown rice (tofu, whole grains) with sprinkling of wheat germ

Lunch: Tossed leafy greens and broccoli salad

Snack: Seeds and Nuts

Dinner: *Black Bean Enchiladas* (kelp, garlic, whole grains), *Yams with Lime* (yams)

Breakfast: *Banana Wheat Germ Muffins* (wheat germ, whole grains)

Lunch: *Onion Tomato Soup* garnished with seeds and nuts

Snack: *Yam Fries*

Dinner: *Fettucine with Garlic* (garlic, whole grains) served on a bed of steamed leafy greens, cruciferous vegetables, and plain diced tofu

Breakfast: *Breakfast Couscous* (whole grains, nuts) sprinkled with wheat germ
Lunch: *Ratatouille* (kelp) over a bed of alfalfa and diced tofu
Snack: *Seed Focaccia* (seeds)
Dinner: *Rice and Feta Sauté* (garlic, broccoli, whole grains); *Yam Salad* (yams)

Breakfast: *Whole Wheat Fruit Bread* (whole grains, nuts, seeds, wheat germ)
Lunch: *Arugula Orange Salad* (greens, nuts); Roast Yams with *Black Soybean Hummus*
Dinner: *Chili* (garlic, kelp) over bed of steamed cruciferous vegetables

Breakfast: *Yam Pancakes* (yams), topped with apple sauce and sprinkled with wheat germ
Lunch: *Mushroom Soup* (kelp, garlic, whole grains); *Kale-Apple Salad with Almonds* (greens, nuts)
Snack: *Pumpkin Seed Brittle*
Dinner: *Indonesian Tofu* (tofu, broccoli, alfalfa, garlic)

Yams

Remember that sweet potatoes and yams are not interchangeable. True yams, of the tuber family known as "Dioscorea," can be purchased in whole foods and health food stores.

Cranberry Yams

This dish is yummy as is, or for more fertility points, top with a smattering of toasted almonds or walnuts.

6 yams
1 cup jellied cranberry sauce
1 cup fresh cranberries
¾ cup orange juice
½ cup honey or maple syrup
1 tsp. grated orange rind
¾ tsp. cinnamon
dash cloves

Boil yams in their skin until barely tender. Peel and slice thickly. Place in oiled baking dish.

In a saucepan, combine the remaining ingredients. Bring to a boil, reduce the heat and simmer for five minutes. Pour over potatoes.

Bake, uncovered, in a preheated 350-degree oven for 20 minutes. Serves 6.

Yam Fries

These are a spicy alternative to French fries. They are tasty on their own, or dress them up as an hors d'ouevre by serving them on a platter with mustard.

4 yams
2 tbs. olive oil
1 tsp. salt
1 tsp. pepper
1 tsp. curry powder
½ tsp. cayenne pepper

In a bowl, combine olive oil, salt, pepper, curry, and cayenne pepper. Mix well.

Cut potatoes into ¼ inch strips. Stir into oil and spice mixture until evenly coated.

Spread on a cookie sheet and bake at 375 degrees for 20 minutes or until tender. Serve hot.

Roast Yams with Apple Juice

This is a satisfying, and simple way to get in a quick yam fix.

3 cups apple juice
2 turnips, peeled and in bite-sized chunks
2 parsnips, peeled and in bite-sized chunks
8 carrots, peeled and sliced
6 yams, peeled, in bite-sized chunks

Boil apple juice about 30 minutes, until reduced to 1 cup.

Place vegetables into large roasting pan. Pour apple juice over vegetables and toss to coat. Roast in 400 degree oven until vegetables are tender and just turning brown, about 45 minutes. Serves 8.

Yam Soup

Cilantro adds a zippy flavor to this rich broth. Roasting the yams brings out a deeper flavor in this dish.

6 yams, peeled and sliced
4 cups skim milk
2 Tbs. cilantro
olive oil

Roast yam slices on a cookie sheet in a 400 degree oven for 20 minutes, until brown. Turn slices over and roast ten more minutes until tender.

Simmer two cups of milk and cilantro over low heat for ten minutes. Add to yams in food processor, and puree until smooth. Return mixture to saucepan, and simmer with remaining milk. Serves 4.

Tsimmes

The combination of cooked yams, prunes, and carrots is a traditional Jewish favorite, good for holiday meals or anytime. This dish reheats well, so I double the portions and plan for leftovers.

½ lb. pitted prunes
6 carrots, peeled and sliced
3 yams, peeled and in chunks
5 Tbs. honey
½ tsp. each of cinnamon and salt
1 Tbs. lemon juice
1/3 cup orange juice

Mix all the ingredients together and bake in a 3-quart casserole, at 300 degrees, for 1-2 hours until vegetables are soft. Serves 8.

Yams with Walnuts

Combines the fertility nutrients of yams with that of walnuts for a double-whammy of a dish.

4 yams
1 cup water
½ cup walnuts, chopped and toasted
dash of salt and pepper
bit of butter

Scrub the yams and roast on a cookie sheet in a 350 degree oven for one hour. Cool.

Scoop out yams and transfer to bowl. Mash with butter, and season with salt and pepper. Scoop back into skins. Sprinkle with chopped walnuts. Serves 4.

Yam Muffins

These take only minutes to make, and are perfect for quick breakfasts or light dessert. They keep well for a few days, so I double this recipe to make sure we will not run out.

1 yam, peeled and baked until very tender
2 eggs, beaten
½ cup milk
½ cup maple syrup or molasses
3 Tbs. butter, melted
1½ cups whole wheat flour
2 tsp. baking powder
1 tsp. cinnamon
few dashes of salt

Mash yam with fork until very smooth. Combine with eggs, milk, maple syrup, and butter. Stir remaining ingredients in gently, just until mixed. Divide into 12 muffin cups. Bake 25 minutes at 400 degrees. Makes 12 muffins.

Yam Puree

Yam Puree is good plain, or you can bake it in individual pie shells for a fancier look. I often make up a few batches of the filling to freeze; then I just defrost and pop into pie shells as I need it.

6 yams, peeled and baked until very tender
1 cup orange juice
3 Tbs. unsalted butter, in bits
2 Tbs. maple syrup
dash of salt and pepper

Mash the yams with a fork until smooth. Add the orange juice, butter, and maple syrup, and heat in a saucepan over low heat, stirring constantly. Season with a dash of salt and pepper. Serves 6.

Yam Salad

A hearty, refreshing change from boring potato salad. This is an easy dish to whip up for unexpected guests and serve alongside a plain tossed salad.

6 yams
2 tbs. non-fat mayonnaise
salt to taste

Boil yams in their skin until tender. Slice into chunks. In a bowl mix with mayonnaise and salt. Good hot or at room temperature. Serves 6.

Alternative: Substitute balsamic vinegar for the mayonnaise for a zingy taste treat.

Yam Slaw

This is a coleslaw-like dish with the tangy flavors of cumin and scallion.   I like it hot or cold, and it often goes into my husband's lunchbox.

4 yams, peeled and shredded
2 Tbs. olive oil
1 tsp. cumin
½ cup scallion, chopped finely
squirt of lemon juice

In a skillet, heat olive oil over high heat until hot. Sauté yams with cumin for two minutes, stirring constantly, until tender. Remove from heat and add scallions and lemon juice. Serves 4.

Yam Chickpea Soup

A yummy treat for a cold winter's day, yam soup also freezes well. Make up a big batch and freeze in individual portions.

3 Tbs. olive oil
4 cups chopped onion
4 cloves finely chopped garlic
4 cups yams, in bite-sized chunks
2 cups diced fresh tomatoes or canned tomato
2 cups chopped green beans
3 cups cooked chickpeas
6 cups water
2 tsp. paprika
1 tsp. cayenne
1 tsp. turmeric
1 tsp. salt
1 tsp. cinnamon

Sauté onions, garlic, and yams in a pot for 20 minutes. Add spices and water. Simmer another 20 minutes. Add remaining ingredients and simmer for 20 more minutes, or until vegetables are tender. Serves 8.

Yam Chili

This is a traditional chili with added sweetness from the yams. A crowd pleaser, it goes well with any of the plain broccoli dishes.

2 Tbs. olive oil
2 onions, in bite-sized chunks
4 tsp. chili powder
2 cups water
2 yams, peeled, in bite-sized chunks
16 oz. stewed tomatoes
1 cup cooked pinto beans, drained
5 Tbs. fresh cilantro, chopped
3 tsp. orange peel, grated

Sauté onions in olive oil over medium heat for five minutes. Add chili powder, water, and yams. Cover pan and simmer gently for ten minutes, until yam is tender. Add tomatoes and beans. Simmer uncovered ten minutes until yam is very tender. Add cilantro and orange peel. Serves 4

Yam Pancakes

These pancakes are reminiscent of Hanukah latkes, only sweeter. They are delectable with applesauce or non-fat sour cream. They are popular around here for breakfasts or mid-afternoon snacks.

2 cups carrots, grated
2 cups white potatoes, grated
2 cups yams, grated
3 eggs, beaten
2/3 cup whole wheat flour
4 Tbs. onion, grated
2 cloves garlic, crushed
2 tsp. salt
dash of black pepper
juice of half a lemon
touch of olive oil

In a colander, place yams, white potatoes, and a touch of salt, and let drain for 20 minutes. Rinse and squeeze out excess water.

Combine all ingredients. In a skillet, fry in olive oil until golden. Serve immediately. Serves 8.

Curried Yam Latkes

In this version of yam latkes, curry adds the zing. These are better as dinner food, served with something crisp and somewhat bland, like a cauliflower salad.

1 lb. yams, peeled and grated coarsely
½ cup whole wheat flour
3 tsp. maple sugar or molasses
½ tsp. cayenne
2 tsp. curry powder
dash of salt and pepper
2 eggs, beaten
½ cup milk
olive oil

In a bowl, mix the flour, eggs, molasses, cayenne, curry, salt and pepper. Add milk until the batter turns slightly stiff. Add the yams. If the batter is now too stiff, add more milk.

Heat the olive oil in a skillet. Use a spoon to drop the batter in and flatten with a spatula. Fry for several minutes on each side, over medium heat, until golden brown. Drain on paper towels and serve warm. Makes 15 latkes.

Cheesy Yams

Cut into wedges, this pie is wonderful comfort food.   Serve it with a nice bean-filled soup on a cold winter's day.

olive oil
4 medium yams, in paper-thin slices
4 Tbs. Parmesan cheese, grated
dash of salt
hint of black pepper

Layer half the yam slices in circles in a greased cake pan. Sprinkle on half the Parmesan and salt and pepper. Place the rest of the potato slices decoratively in the pan, and finish with the cheese and seasonings. Cover with foil.

Bake 45 minutes in a 400 degree oven.   Uncover and bake another 30 minutes, until tender.   Let sit five minutes before serving.

Yam Croquettes

Yam croquettes are an addictive snack. For party appetizers I make little bite-sized croquettes and serve them with dipping sauces.

5 yams, peeled, cut into chunks
1/3 cup molasses or maple syrup
½ tsp. vanilla extract
1 egg
½ cup cornflake crumbs or breadcrumbs
1 cup whole wheat flour
olive oil

Steam yams 15 minutes until tender. Place in bowl with molasses, vanilla, eggs, and crumbs, and mash well.

Shape yam mixture into tablespoon-sized balls and coat in flour. Place on tinfoil-lined baking sheet.

Heat olive oil until very hot. Fry croquettes in batches for five minutes, until golden brown. Drain on paper towels. Makes 15.

Yams with Lime

This is the easiest way to cook and serve yams, and for me, the tastiest. These taste like they were fussed over.

4 medium yams
some olive oil
juice of 2 limes

Scrub the yams and rub with olive oil. Puncture the skins with a fork. Bake for 50-60 minutes until tender.

Slit open and mash into each potato half some lime juice. Serves 4.

Yam and Apple Casserole

This casserole combines the tartness of apple with the sweetness of yam. It also provides extra sunflower seeds, almonds, and wheat germ.

2 apples, cored and diced
juice of half a lime
4 medium yams, peeled and sliced
1/3 cup raisins
½ cup sunflower seeds or sliced almonds, or a combination
1/3 cup wheat germ
2 cups apple cider
2 Tbs. honey
½ tsp. each allspice, cinnamon, and mace
dash of salt

In a bowl, toss the apples, lime juice, yams, raisins, wheat germ and sunflower seeds or almonds.

In a saucepan, gently heat the cider, honey, salt and spices. Pour over the yam-apple mixture and toss.

Place in a buttered 2 quart casserole dish, cover, and bake for 1 hour until tender. Serve hot. Serves 6.

Curried Yams

These are quite simple to make, but oh-so-good.

2 Tbs. olive oil
2 tsp. curry powder
4 cups yams, peeled, in bite-sized chunks
dash of salt and pepper

In a saucepan, heat curry powder, salt and pepper in olive oil. Toss with yams. In 450 degree oven, roast yams 20 minutes until tender and golden brown. Serves 4.

Green Yam Salad

This is a colorful side dish that goes particularly well with fish, and is packed full of fertility nutrients.

6 yams, peeled, in chunks
3 Tbs. mustard
3 Tbs. honey
1 bunch Swiss Chard, trimmed, in bite-sized pieces
olive oil

Steam yams for ten minutes, until tender. Cool

In a large skillet over medium heat, sauté Swiss Chard in olive oil two minutes, until barely wilted. Add yams, mustard, and honey. Heat for another two minutes. Serves 6.

Fruited Yam Casserole

An incredibly satisfying dish that is based on a recipe by Martha Rose Shulman, one of my favorite cookbook authors. I serve it as dessert for our large annual Thanksgiving dinner, and it is invariably more popular than the apple pies and chocolate brownies.

3 yams, peeled
½ cup honey
½ cup slivered almonds or sunflower seeds or both
2 tsp. cinnamon
2 apples, cored and sliced
½ cup raisins
3 bananas, sliced
dash of orange juice

Steam the yam about 20 minutes until tender. Drain and slice. Arrange the slices in a 2-quart oiled baking dish. Brush with some of the honey. Combine apples, raisins, seeds, nuts and cinnamon, and layer on top. Brush with some more honey. Layer banana slices over the top. Cover with orange juice, and sprinkle with a little more cinnamon.

Bake in 350 degree oven for 45 minutes until the bananas are turning brown. Serve hot. Serves 6.

Garlic

Walnut Risotto with Garlic

This is a time-consuming dish to make, but a yummy one. Besides the garlic, it contains brown rice and walnuts, making it a powerhouse of fertility foods.

5 cups water or vegetable stock
3 tsp. olive oil
½ cup onion, chopped
1½ cups brown rice
1 lb. asparagus
2 garlic cloves, thinly sliced
¼ cup walnuts, finely chopped and toasted
2 Tbs. fresh Parmesan cheese, grated

In a skillet, sauté onion in olive oil until golden. Add rice and stir for three minutes. Add ½ cup water or vegetable stock and cook until liquid is absorbed, stirring frequently. Continue adding more stock, half a cup at a time, until rice is creamy. Stir frequently and allow the stock to be absorbed before adding more. This whole process should take about half an hour.

Meanwhile, place asparagus and garlic in a shallow baking dish and drizzle with olive oil. Bake about 15-20 minutes until tender. Place in center of serving platter.

Mix walnuts and Parmesan into risotto. Arrange on top of asparagus and garlic. Serves 4.

Garlic Dressing

This is a nice topping for leafy greens or whole wheat pasta.

½ cup mayonnaise
½ cup plain, nonfat yogurt
3 garlic cloves, crushed
1 tsp. mustard
2 Tbs. lemon juice

Mix the mayonnaise and yogurt until smooth. Add the garlic, mustard, and lemon juice until well blended.   Chill. Makes 1 cup.

Garlic Hummus

Hummus is a family favorite; easy to make and always satisfyingly filling. We serve it as dip with veggies, and take it in pita sandwiches off to lunch.

3 garlic cloves, crushed
18 oz. chickpeas, drained
1/3 cup tahini
2 Tbs. lemon juice
2 Tbs. olive oil
dash of cumin
dash of salt

Blend the garlic, chickpeas, tahini, lemon juice, oil, and cumin until smooth. Add a splash of water and salt. Serves 4.

Tuna Nicoise with Garlic

This is a garlicky, Mediterranean variant on traditional tuna nicoise. It is laden with leafy greens and almonds as well as the garlic: a fertility powerhouse.

¼ cup olive oil
¼ cup balsamic vinegar
3 Tbs. garlic, crushed
3 oranges, in segments, seeds removed
1 onion, sliced
1 red pepper, sliced
1 avocado, in bite-sized chunks
9 oz. white tuna, drained
7 cups leafy salad greens
1/3 cup almonds, toasted

Whisk oil, vinegar, and garlic together. Add orange segments, onion, pepper, avocado, and tuna. Spoon over platter of salad greens. Garnish with almonds. Serves 4.

Garlic Tofu Pate

This is an easy, nice lunch spread, containing not only garlic but lots of tofu besides. Try it in a whole wheat pita with lots of leafy greens.

½ lb. firm tofu
2 garlic cloves, crushed
2 tsp. soy sauce
dash of oregano and dill

Blend the tofu, garlic, and tamari until smooth. Stir in the herbs, and chill at least 30 minutes.

Garlic Lentil Soup

This is a full-bodied soup with a nice tangy taste. Ladle it over a mound of brown rice and steamed greens.

¼ cup olive oil
6 garlic cloves, crushed
3 onions, in chunks
8 cups water
1 cup lentils
4 carrots, peeled and sliced
¼ cup tomato paste mixed with ½ cup water
1 Tbs. soy sauce
dash of salt and pepper

Sauté the garlic and onions in olive oil ten minutes, until golden, stirring often. Add the remaining ingredients. Bring to a boil, then reduce to a simmer for 45 minutes. Serves 4.

Good Old Garlic Soup

This is a wonderful garlic soup on which to base a more elaborate soup or stew, or enjoy as is.

2 heads garlic, peeled
2 quarts vegetable stock or water
2 tsp. salt
dash of pepper
2 cloves
2 Tbs. olive oil

Bring the garlic, vegetable stock, salt, pepper, cloves, and oil to a gentle boil. Lower heat and simmer for one hour. Strain out the garlic and cloves. Serves 6.

Garlic-Eggplant Puree

This is a simple, wonderful dish, based on a recipe by Deborah Madison.

1 eggplant
2 cloves garlic, thinly sliced
grated peel and juice of 1 lemon
1 Tbs. olive oil
1 tsp. cilantro
1 Tbs. plain unsweetened yogurt
dash of salt and pepper
a few cilantro leaves for garnish

With a sharp knife, make incisions all over the eggplant and insert a sliver of garlic into each one. Bake the eggplant about 1 hour, until thoroughly wrinkled. Drain in a colander for 30 minutes.

After it has drained, scrape the meat and garlic slivers out of the eggplant skin. Chop it finely to make a coarse puree. Stir in the lemon peel, olive oil, cilantro, and yogurt. Season with lemon juice, salt, and pepper. Mound it in a bowl, and garnish with whole cilantro leaves. Serves 2.

Caramelized Potato Garlic Pie

This is a lovely caramelized casserole, and one of the very few recipes where I am not tempted to substitute yams!

6 potatoes, thinly sliced
3 onions, thinly sliced
5 garlic cloves, crushed
28 oz. crushed plum tomatoes, drained
¼ cup tomato paste
½ cup olive oil
3 Tbs. water
2 tsp. oregano
dash of salt and pepper

Mix the tomato paste, olive oil, water, oregano, salt and pepper in a large bowl. Add the potatoes, onions, garlic, and tomatoes and mix well. Pour into an oiled baking dish and cover. Bake 30 minutes at 400 degrees. Remove cover and bake another 45 minutes, until potatoes are tender. Serves 4.

Garlic Tomato Sauce

This is nice over whole grain noodles or steamed greens.

2 Tbs. olive oil
1 onion, chopped
3 cloves garlic, crushed
1 Tbs. whole wheat flour
1 tsp. paprika
15 oz. crushed tomatoes, drained; reserve juice
dash of pepper

Sauté onion and garlic in olive oil until onion is softened. Stir in flour and paprika; cook for one minute. Stir in reserved liquid from tomatoes. Cook, stirring constantly, for two minutes until sauce thickens.

Add tomatoes and pepper. Stir until warm. Serves two.

Fettucine with Garlic

This is garlic lover's heaven, with whole wheat pasta to boot. You can also add steamed broccoli and cauliflower to up your day's intake of cruciferous vegetables.

1 lb. zucchini, cut into strips
1/3 cup olive oil
4 tsp. garlic, crushed
¾ lb. whole wheat fettucine
½ cup Parmesan cheese
dash of salt and pepper

Steam the zucchini for five minutes. Meanwhile, cook the pasta.

Sauté the garlic in olive oil over very low heat, for about ten minutes, until it turns golden. Toss with the cooked pasta, and add the remaining ingredients.   Garnish with Parmesan. Serves 4.

Couscous Garlic Salad

This is a pretty and appetizing combination.   Better yet, it requires little cooking!

1½ cups couscous
½ cup raisins
1 tsp. turmeric
2 cups boiling water
1 cup almonds, slivered
2 cups cooked chickpeas, drained
2 scallions, sliced
2 medium tomatoes, in bite-sized chunks
1/3 cup lemon juice
1/3 cup olive oil
3 garlic cloves, crushed
grated rind of 1 orange
sprinkling of wheat germ
dash of salt and pepper

Pour boiling water over the couscous, raisins and turmeric. Stir and cover with a plate for fifteen minutes.

Stir in the chickpeas, almonds, scallions, and tomatoes.

Combine the lemon juice, olive oil, garlic, orange rind, wheat germ, and salt and pepper. Toss over the couscous. Chill 30 minutes. Serves 4.

Garlic Butter

Despite seriously curtailing our butter consumption, this recipe remains one of the few holdouts, for one reason: It is amazing, and incredibly simple. Do not eat it too often.

½ cup butter
garlic, crushed - as much as you can tolerate
optional herbs: chives and dill are my favorites

Mix the butter and garlic together thoroughly, and serve with warm whole wheat bread. Mmmm!

Picnic Bean and Garlic Salad

This is our favorite vegetable dish for a summer picnic or potluck supper. Besides the garlic, it is full of almonds.

¼ cup almonds
4 tsp. soy sauce
1 lb. green beans, in bite-sized pieces
2 Tbs. rice vinegar
2 large garlic cloves, crushed
2 Tbs. green onions, sliced
1/3 cup cilantro

Sauté almonds in a skillet five minutes, until lightly toasted. Add 3 tsp. soy sauce and stir until almonds are coated. Cool. Chop almonds.

Cook green beans in boiling water five minutes, until tender. Drain and rinse. Refrigerate beans for half hour.

Whisk vinegar, oil, garlic, and remaining soy sauce in a bowl. Coat green beans thoroughly.   Sprinkle green onions, cilantro, and almonds on top. Serves 4.

Tofu and Black Soybeans

Tofu Chowder

This is a creamy chowder reminiscent of cream soups but healthier for you. It is nice with a big plate of spicy greens.

1 onion, in bite-sized chunks
1 Tbs. olive oil
1 tsp. whole wheat flour
1 cup garlic soup stock or water
1 cup cucumber, peeled, in bite-sized chunks
1 cup silken tofu, drained
2 tsp. lemon juice
2 Tbs. fresh dill, minced

Sauté the onions in olive oil over low heat, until soft. Add flour, broth, and cucumber, and bring to a boil.

Puree the mixture with the tofu and lemon juice until smooth. Stir in the dill. Serves 2.

Corn Tofu Chowder

This is another tofu-based chowder, with corn for a southwest taste. The optional turmeric gives it a little extra kick. In the morning we heat up the leftovers and ladle over cooked brown rice or barley for a comforting, unusual breakfast porridge.

6 ears fresh corn, shucked
8 cups water
1 lb. silken tofu, drained
1 cup scallions, sliced
dash of salt and pepper
optional: ½ tsp. turmeric
dash of cumin

Cut kernels off cobs, reserving cobs. In a large pot, simmer water, corn, cobs, and salt and pepper, uncovered, 20 minutes. Discard corn cobs.

In batches, puree tofu with corn mixture until smooth. Return to pot. Stir in scallions, turmeric (and cumin if desired) and heat through. Serves 6.

Tofu Hot and Sour Soup

This is another nice tofu-heavy soup, with some tasty touches from the far east.

1 oz. dried shiitake mushrooms, rinsed
8 cups water
½ cup cider vinegar
2 Tbs. tamari
dash of salt
1 lb. firm tofu, sliced in thin strips
5 minced scallions
dash of pepper
dash of turmeric

Pour two cups boiling water over shiitake mushrooms and let stand 30 minutes. Then slice mushrooms and discard stems.

Heat mushroom water and remaining water to boiling. Add vinegar, tamari, salt, mushrooms, and tofu. Simmer ten minutes. Add scallions, turmeric and pepper, and cook two more minutes. Serves 6.

Tofu Dressing

This makes a versatile and easy dip, salad dressing, or fish garnish. It is a really quick, "Uh oh, it's dinner time and there is no food in the house" sort of dish.

1 lb. soft or silken tofu, drained
3 Tbs. mustard
1 Tbs. lemon juice
1 garlic clove
dash of turmeric
1 bunch fresh chives, minced

Puree everything but the chives until smooth.   Stir in chives.
Makes 1 cup.

Tuna Tofu Dip

This is another quick dip that goes well with vegetables or even as a sandwich spread.

12 oz. white tuna, drained
1 lb. soft or silken tofu, drained
2 scallions, minced
2 carrots, shredded
2 Tbs. capers, drained
3 Tbs. lemon juice.

Whisk tofu until smooth. Stir in tuna and remaining ingredients until thoroughly combined. Makes 3 cups.

Tofu with Garlic Sauce

This is a fast and elegant supper with an Oriental flavor.

1 lb. firm tofu
1 cup water
2 Tbs. soy sauce
1 Tbs. cider vinegar
2 tsp. molasses or maple syrup
dash of salt
2 Tbs. olive oil
4 garlic cloves, minced
1 tsp. sesame oil
1 scallion

Place the tofu under a cookie tray with a weight on top so it will drain for 30 minutes. Meantime, sauté the garlic in 1½ Tbs. olive oil for one minute. Add in the soy sauce, vinegar, molasses, salt, and water, stirring, and bring to a boil. Simmer for two minutes and stir in the sesame oil.

In another skillet, sauté the drained tofu in the remaining olive oil until brown. Drain on paper towels to remove oil, and then drizzle with sauce. Garnish with scallion. Serves 2.

Potatoes Masala

We become addicted to this dish while traveling in India. This is a healthier version of it than the one we consumed; it is also easier to prepare.   We've substituted greenbeans for the traditional peas that are a fertility no-no.

3 Tbs. olive oil
2 onion, in chunks
30 oz. canned tomatoes
2 potatoes, in bite-sized chunks
2 tsp. cumin
1 tsp. allspice
1 lb. firm tofu, drained, in bite-sized chunks
5 cups green beans, chopped
5 Tbs. cilantro, chopped
dash of turmeric

Sauté onion in olive oil five minutes. Add tomatoes, potatoes, cumin and allspice. Cover and simmer ten minutes. Add tofu, green beans, cilantro and turmeric. Simmer uncovered five minutes, until potatoes are tender. Serves 4.

Tofu Potato Salad

Here, the tofu provides a creamy mayonnaise for the potato salad. This keeps for a few days in the refrigerator.

12 baby red potatoes, scrubbed
1 lb. soft tofu
2 Tbs. lemon juice
2 Tbs. water
2 Tbs. olive oil
1 red onion, sliced
dash of salt and pepper

Boil the potatoes in water for 20 minutes until tender; then drain. Meanwhile, blend the tofu, lemon juice, and water until just combined. Add the olive oil in a stream slowly and continue to blend.

Toss the potatoes with onion, mayonnaise, and salt and pepper. Serves 4.

Black Soybean Nibbles

This is great for munchfood at parties and in front of the television set. We have taken to smuggling it into movie theaters so we are not tempted by the greasy popcorn.

2 Tbs. olive oil
dash of cayenne, cumin, and turmeric
2 cups unseasoned dry-roasted black soybeans
1 cup freeze-dried greenbeans or chickpeas

Quickly sauté the cayenne, cumin, and turmeric in olive oil, about ten seconds. Add soybeans and vegetables, tossing to combine. Cool on paper towels. Store in sealed jar at room temperature.

Tofu Stir Fry

There are many variations of tofu stir fry. This one uses yellow squash and cheese to make this true comfort food.

3 Tbs. olive oil
1 lb. firm tofu, drained and cut into cubes
2 onions, in chunks
2 yellow squash, sliced
½ cup tomato sauce
1 cup cheddar or Muenster cheese, grated
dash of pepper

Stir fry the tofu in olive oil for ten minutes, until golden. Remove from pan. In the same pan, sauté the onions and squash for ten minutes. Then add the tofu back in, along with the tomato sauce, and sauté for three more minutes. Sprinkle on the pepper and cheese, and cook, covered, for two more minutes. Serves 4.

Indonesia Tofu

This recipe is very loosely based on one I first saw in Molly Katzen's "Moosewood" Cookbook, still the best cookbook there is.

1 lb. firm tofu, in bite-sized chunks
fresh vegetables of your choice: carrot, broccoli, alfalfa
1 cup onion, chopped
3 cloves garlic, crushed
1 cup peanut butter
1 Tbs. honey
dash of cayenne
juice of 1 lemon
1 Tbs. cider vinegar
3 cups water
dash of salt
olive oil

Arrange vegetables and tofu on platter.

Sauté the onions and garlic in olive oil for five minutes. Add remaining ingredients and simmer on low heat for 30 minutes, stirring occasionally.   Drizzle over tofu-vegetable platter. Serves 6.

Black Soybean Hummus

A version of hummus, this one with the nutty addition of black soybeans, a Macrobiotic favorite for fertility enhancement.

2 cloves garlic, peeled
3 cups black soybeans, cooked and drained
4 Tbs. lemon juice
5 Tbs. soybean cooking water
3 Tbs. tahini
dash of salt, cayenne, and turmeric

Puree to a paste in a food processor the garlic and black soybeans. Add the remaining ingredients and blend until smooth. Serves 4.

Kelp

Although kelp is not considered a common ingredient in this part of the world, it is really very easy to use. In addition to the recipes described here, try adding a one-inch piece of kelp anytime you are cooking a soup, stock, chili, or stew. Simply add the kelp to the cooking water. In dishes that must be pureed, remove the kelp before pureeing. In other dishes, simply discard the kelp before serving. Kelp helps soups and stews cook faster, and when used in bean dishes, makes the beans more tender and helps minimize their gassy tendencies.

"Beef" Stock

This completely vegetable stock has a rich, "beef-like" flavor. Make a big batch and freeze in portions. It is tasty as is, or use it as the basis for a more elaborate soup or stew.

2 quarts water
2 onions, in chunks
2 carrots, peeled, in chunks
2 stalks celery, in chunks
3 potatoes, unpeeled, in large chunks
2 leeks, white part only, in chunks
6 cloves garlic
dash of salt and pepper
1 Tbs. tamari
2 tsp. miso
1 inch piece of kelp

Combine all ingredients in a soup pot and bring to a gentle boil. Reduce heat and simmer uncovered for 2 hours.

Strain and discard vegetables and kelp. Makes 2 quarts.

Sweet "Beef" Stock

This is another faux beef stock, with an added depth of sweetness because of the yams. Again, it works as a soup on its own, or as a basis for a more elaborate soup.

2 quarts water
2 onions, in chunks
2 carrots, peeled, in chunks
3 yams or yams, unpeeled, in large chunks
2 leeks, white part only, in chunks
6 cloves garlic
dash of salt and pepper
1 Tbs. tamari
2 tsp. Marmite or miso
1 inch piece of kelp

Combine all ingredients in a soup pot and bring to a gentle boil. Reduce heat and simmer uncovered for 2 hours.

Strain and discard vegetables and kelp. Makes 2 quarts.

Ratatouille

This is a tomato-based vegetable stew, good hot or cold. Serve it as a side dish or as stuffing for an omelet or pepper. The leftovers disappear into lunchboxes, so you might want to double the recipe...

1 eggplant, washed and in bite-sized chunks
¼ cup olive oil
2 onions in chunks
4 cloves garlic, crushed
2 zucchini, in chunks
2 yellow squash, in chunks
½ cup tomato paste
½ cup water
4 tomatoes, in chunks
2 tsp. oregano
dash of salt and pepper
1 inch piece of kelp

Sauté the onion and garlic in olive oil for five minutes. Add the eggplant, zucchini, and yellow squash, and stir well.

Add the tomato paste, water, tomato, spices and kelp and cook over low heat for 1 hour. Discard kelp. Serves 6.

Mushroom Soup

This is a deep, flavorful soup that is a perennial crowd pleaser.
It also contains garlic and whole wheat bread.

2 Tbs. butter or olive oil
1 onion, diced
dash of salt
2 garlic cloves, in chunks
1 lb. mushrooms, in chunks
6 cups vegetable stock or water
1 inch piece of kelp
2 slices whole wheat bread
½ cup light cream
dash of pepper
optional: chives for garnish

Sauté the onion and salt in butter or olive oil for 3 minutes.
Add the garlic and cook two more minutes.   Add the
mushrooms and continue sautéing for 8 minutes, stirring
occasionally. Add the water and kelp and bring to a boil. Add
the bread and simmer for 20 minutes. Cool. Discard kelp.

Puree the soup until desired degree of creamy. Reheat, and stir
in the cream and pepper. Serves 4.

Chili

The addition of kelp to this hearty chili recipe eliminates the gassy effects of the beans. It is yummy.

8 tomatoes
2 Tbs. olive oil
2 onions, in chunks
4 cloves garlic, crushed
15 oz. tomato sauce
4 cups pinto or kidney beans, cooked and drained
1 inch piece of kelp
1 Tbs. chili powder
1 Tbs. cumin
optional: 2 Tbs. cilantro, chopped
optional: handful of raisins

Sauté the onions and garlic in olive oil until tender. Add beans, tomatoes, tomato sauce, spices, and kelp. Cover and simmer for one hour, stirring occasionally. Discard kelp. Serves 6.

Creamy Garlic Potato Soup

This is a wonderfully rich, creamy soup—without cream! It is the potato that gives it its body. And you get extra fertility points for the garlic.

1 Tbs. olive oil
1 onion, in chunks
1 head garlic, peeled
6 stalks celery, sliced
1 large potato, peeled and in chunks
8 cups water or vegetable stock
1 inch piece of kelp
dash of salt and pepper

Sauté the onion in olive oil three minutes. Add the garlic and celery and sauté another two minutes. Add the potato, water, and kelp and bring to a simmer. Cover and simmer for 30 minutes. Add a dash of salt and pepper. Remove kelp and discard. Puree soup until smooth. Heat through. Serves 6.

Onion Tomato Soup

A wonderfully soothing soup, try serving it over a chunk of French bread with a bit of melting cheese. It is also good with whole wheat bread or brown rice and toasted seeds as garnish.

4 onions, in chunks
2 cloves garlic, crushed
3 Tbs. olive oil
1 quart vegetable stock or water
2 cups tomato juice
1 inch piece of kelp
dash of tarragon
2 tsp. lemon juice
dash of salt and pepper

Sauté the onions and garlic in olive oil for a few minutes. Add the water, tomato juice, kelp, tarragon, lemon juice, and salt and pepper. Cover and simmer for one hour. Discard the kelp. Serves 6.

Tomato Potato Soup

A nice winter soup that is fast and easy to prepare.

2 onions, in chunks
3 Tbs. olive oil
2 potatoes, in chunks
1 quart vegetable stock or water
1 inch piece of kelp
5 cups tomatoes, sliced
1 tsp. honey
dash of salt and paprika
1 cup milk or cream

Sauté the onion in olive oil for a few minutes. Add the potatoes, water and kelp. Cover and simmer for 30 minutes.

Add the tomatoes, honey, salt and paprika and simmer for another 30 minutes. Discard the kelp.

Puree some of the soup or all of the soup, if desired. Then stir in the milk or cream. Heat through on very low heat so the milk will not curdle. Serves 6.

Black Bean Enchiladas

Once the beans are cooked, this dish takes very little time to prepare, but it looks as though it has taken all day! A scrumptious meal, sure to be a family favorite.

2 cups dried black beans
1 inch piece of kelp
6 cups water
2 Tbs. olive oil
1 onion, in chunks
5 cloves garlic, crushed
1 Tbs. cumin
1 Tbs. chili powder
dash of salt
12 corn tortillas
½ onion, finely diced
3 tomatoes, diced
2 avocados, diced
12 oz. cheese (cheddar or even American), in chunks
3 cups salsa, mild
optional: 2 cups cooked brown rice

Soak the beans and kelp in water for several hours. When the beans are soaked, sauté the onion and garlic in olive oil for 3 minutes. Add the soaked beans and their water, and the kelp, and bring to a boil. Cover and simmer for 2-3 hours, until the beans are very soft. Drain off the cooking water and discard the kelp. Mix in the cumin, chili powder, and salt and stir. If desired, puree some of the beans.

Splash some salsa on the inside of a lasagna-sized baking pan. Place the corn tortillas in the pan. Fill each tortilla with the optional rice, a scoop or two of black beans, some tomatoes, a bit of onion, a little avocado, and a sprinkling of cheese.. Top each tortilla with another splash of salsa. Bake at 350 degrees for 40 minutes. Serves 6.

Whole Grains

Balinese Rice

We discovered this style of rice preparation while in Indonesia, where all the food looks (and tastes) beautiful. An easy way to spiff up plain brown rice beyond recognition.

4 cups water
2 cups brown rice
½ cup raisins
1 onion, in small chunks
3 cloves garlic, crushed
1 Tbs. olive oil
1/3 cup almonds, slivered
optional: ½ cup chutney, any kind
dash of salt

Boil the water and add the rice.   Simmer, covered for 35 minutes until all the water is absorbed.

After the rice is cooked, sauté the onions and garlic in olive oil for ten minutes.   Add the raisins, almonds, and chutney if desired. After five minutes, stir in the cooked rice and cook for five more minutes. Serves 6.

Soba Surprise

The surprise is how easy this dish is to make, and how tasty it is. These buckwheat noodles cook faster than spaghetti, with a nutty, grittier flavor. Unlike spaghetti, they are also really good cold. This dish goes well with a salad.

large pot of boiling water
½ lb. soba noodles
3 Tbs. sesame oil
1 Tbs. tamari

Cook the soba noodles in boiling water for just five minutes. Remove quickly and drain. Add the sesame oil and tamari and toss. Serves 6.

Moroccan Couscous

This is a middle eastern dish that is ready in minutes, but looks like you spent a lot more time on it.

3 cups whole wheat couscous
6 cups water, boiling
½ cup almonds, chopped
1 Tbs. olive oil
1 cup onion, in chunks
1 cup carrot, in chunks
1 cup zucchini, in chunks
1½ tsp. cumin
1½ tsp. coriander
1/3 cup raisins
1 cup vegetable stock or water

Pour the boiling water over the couscous and cover for 30 minutes.

Sauté the almonds in olive oil over medium heat for 5 minutes. Remove almonds with slotted spoon.

Sauté vegetables, cumin, and coriander for four minutes. Add raisins and water and simmer for 10 more minutes.

Place the finished couscous on plates, and spoon sautéed vegetables and sauce over it. Garnish with almonds. Serves 6.

Breakfast Couscous

Breakfast couscous can be prepared the night before.   The addition of dates makes this dish particularly lively.

3 cups couscous
6 cups water
½ cup maple syrup
1½ cup almonds, toasted and sliced
8 oz. pitted dates, diced
optional: 2 cups milk

Place couscous in baking dish. In a pot, boil water with maple syrup.   Pour over couscous and cover.   Let stand fifteen minutes.

Mix nuts and dates into couscous. Bake couscous 20 minutes at 350 degrees.   Serve in individual bowls, with milk if desired. Serves 6.

Barley Casserole

Try this as company fare, and listen to the comments! You can also vary this recipe by adding quite a bit more water, and letting it turn into a stew or soup.

2 Tbs. olive oil
2 onions, diced
5 cups mushrooms, diced
1½ cups barley
dash of salt and pepper
5 cups vegetable stock or water

Sauté the onions, mushrooms, barley, salt and pepper in olive oil over medium high for ten minutes.

Transfer to 2-quart casserole dish and add the vegetable stock or water. Cover and bake 75 minutes, until the liquid is absorbed. If the barley is too crunchy, add a bit more water and return to oven for five minutes. Serves 4.

Cranberry Bulgur

An unusual but delectable way to serve bulgur, and very pretty to look at.

3 Tbs. olive oil
3 cups leeks, diced
6 cups vegetable stock or water
3 cups bulgur
2/3 cup dried cranberries
2/3 cup almonds, toasted and sliced

Sauté leeks in olive oil for 15 minutes. Add the water and boil. Stir in the bulgur and cook five minutes.

Remove from the heat and add the dried cranberries. Cover pot and let stand 15 minutes. Mix in almonds. Serves 4.

Curried Barley Soup

A spicy way to dress up barley. You can sprinkle wheat germ or toasted nuts on the top for extra fertility points.

2 Tbs. olive oil
2 onions, diced
2 garlic cloves, crushed
5 cups mushrooms, in chunks
2 tsp. coriander
2 tsp. cumin
1 tsp. turmeric
dash each of cardamom, cayenne, pepper
1 cup barley
7 cups water
dash of salt
1 Tbs. soy sauce
1 inch piece of kelp
optional: ½ cup milk

Sauté the onions and garlic over medium heat for four minutes. Add the mushrooms and sauté another five minutes. Add the spices and stir.

Add the barley and cook three more minutes. Then add the water, salt, and soy sauce, and cover the pot. Simmer for 1 hour, until barley is tender. Discard the kelp.

Remove from the heat and swirl in the milk. Serves 4.

Lentil Bulgur Salad

A wonderful salad for picnics or potlucks: filling, tasty, and easy to make.

½ cup shallots, diced
2 cups water
3 Tbs. balsamic vinegar
½ cup green lentils
1 cup bulgur
dash of salt
½ cup carrot, shredded
3 Tbs. olive oil
½ cup walnuts, toasted and chopped

Simmer lentils in ½ cup water for 20 minutes. Drain well. Add shallots and 1 Tbs. vinegar. Cool.

Simmer bulgur and salt in 1½ cups water, covered, for 15 minutes until all the water is absorbed. Cool.

Combine lentils and bulgur with carrots, the rest of the vinegar, oil, and walnuts, and toss well. Serves 6.

Fern's Chickpea Stew

This is one of my most renowned—and easiest—dishes: True comfort food for a rainy or unhappy day.

4 cups boiling water
2 cups brown rice
2 cups chickpeas, cooked
2 cups canned crushed tomatoes
½ cup raisins
dash of cardamom, cumin, salt and pepper
handful of pumpkin or sunflower seeds

Cook the brown rice, covered, in boiling water for 50 minutes until all the water is absorbed.

Meanwhile, cook the chickpeas, tomatoes, raisins and spices over medium heat for one hour. Ladle over cooked rice. Toss on a sprinkling of sunflower or pumpkin seeds. Serves 4.

Elegant Brown Rice

A fancy way to serve brown rice without fussing.

3 cups water
½ tsp. salt
1½ cup brown rice
½ cup almonds, toasted and slivered
4 Tbs. raisins

Bring water to a boil. Add rice and salt and cook, covered, for 25 minutes over low heat. Stir in almonds and raisins and let stand for 5 minutes. Serves 4.

Tabbouli

This middle eastern dish never ceases to satisfy my craving for sweets and starch. Here, I have taken out the parsley and increased the mint and raisins instead.

2 cups water, boiling
1 cup bulgur
2 onions, in small chunks
2 cup fresh mint leaves, shredded
2 tomatoes, diced
¼ cup olive oil
juice of 2 lemons
dash of salt and pepper

Soak the bulgur in boiling water for 2 hours.

After the bulgur is ready, add everything else and season to taste. Serves 6.

Rice and Feta Sauté

I have seen several variations of this dish; here is my favorite, because of the zing the feta adds. You also benefit from the garlic and broccoli.

4 cups water, boiling
2 cups brown rice
2 Tbs. olive oil
4 garlic cloves, crushed
2 tomatoes, in small chunks
1 bunch broccoli, in bite sized chunks
dash of oregano
½ cup water
1 cup feta cheese, crumbled
dash of pepper

Cook the rice in boiling water, covered, or 50 minutes.

When the rice is cooked, sauté garlic in olive oil for two minutes. Add the tomatoes and sauté two more minutes. Add the broccoli, oregano, and water, and cook, covered, for another five minutes.

Stir in the hot rice, feta cheese, and dash of pepper. Serves 4.

Whole Wheat Quick Lasagna

The secret to this dish is that the lasagna noodles do not need to be precooked.

2 eggs
2 cups skim ricotta cheese
¼ cup parmesan cheese, grated
dash of salt and pepper
4 cups tomato sauce, mixed with 1 cup water
2 cups broccoli, steamed
1 lb. whole-wheat lasagna noodles, uncooked
6 cups mozzarella cheese, grated

Combine the eggs, ricotta, Parmesan cheese, salt and pepper in a bowl. Cover the bottom of a lasagna pan with tomato sauce. Alternate layers of lasagna, sauce, broccoli, ricotta mixture, and grated mozzarella, two or three times. The last time, end up with the mozzarella on the top.

Cover the pan tightly with aluminum foil. Bake 1 hour at 350 degrees. Then remove the tinfoil and bake another ten minutes. Serves 6.

Whole Wheat Fruit Bread

Based on Julie Jordan's Wings of Life Bread, this is a nutty, fruity whole wheat bread—the best there is. You can increase the quantity of nuts if you need to.

4 cups yogurt
4 ripe bananas
½ cup sesame oil
½ cup maple syrup
dash of salt
3 cups walnuts, in chunks
3 cups dried apricots, in chunks
3 cups raisins
½ cup sunflower seeds
1 cup wheat germ
10 cups whole wheat flour

Mix the yogurt, bananas, sesame oil, maple syrup, and salt. Add in the walnuts, apricots, raisins, seeds, wheat germ and flour. Mix with a spoon.

When the dough holds together, knead on your kitchen counter for at least fifteen minutes. Shape the dough into two round loaves. Carve slashes on the top so the crusts will not split while baking. Place on lightly oiled cookie sheets and bake at 350 degrees for 1½ hour until deep brown. This bread can be left unwrapped in your kitchen for several days. Makes two loaves.

Mattar Paneer Over Rice

We discovered this while traveling in northern India, and have not been able to shed our craving for it.   This is a complete meal in itself, although we often serve it with a tossed salad. Again, we have substituted green beans for the traditional peas.

4 cups boiling water
2 cups brown rice
2 potatoes,
2 cups green beans
½ cup water
2 onions, in small chunks
2 Tbs. olive oil
2 tsp. curry powder
3 Tbs. fresh mint, minced; or 1 tsp. dried mint
2 cups cottage cheese

Add the brown rice, and two potatoes, to the boiling water. Cook for 50 minutes, until water is all absorbed.   Remove the potatoes.

When rice is done, steam the green beans in the ½ cup of water. If they were fresh, run them under cold water to preserve their bright color.

Sauté the onion and curry powder in olive oil for five minutes. Then add the cooked beans, potatoes, and mint and cook one more minute.   Remove from the heat and stir in the cottage cheese. Ladle over portions of brown rice. Serves 4.

Cruciferous Vegetables

Cruciferous vegetables are a powerhouse for fertility. In addition to their role in ensuring a healthy uterine lining, and their high calcium content that protects against infertility caused by vitamin D deficiencies, their high doses of Vitamin C, without the detrimental effects of taking supplemental Vitamin C, improve sperm motility, sperm viability, and sperm count. Husbands, eat your broccoli!

And remember that indoles can be deactivated by heat, so do not cook these vegetables to death.

Broccoli Pesto

As soon as I read in the herbal literature that both basil and parsley might be counterproductive for fertility, I stopped making pesto. But I really missed it. After a while, I started making it again—out of broccoli, cilantro, and almost every other green vegetable and herb on the fertility list. Here is one variant made from broccoli; it goes nicely over pasta or vegetables.

large pot of boiling water
7 cups broccoli florets or rabe
¼ cup pine nuts
5 garlic cloves
2 Tbs. olive oil
1 Tbs. white wine vinegar
dash of dried red pepper

Cook broccoli in boiling water about ten minutes.

Puree broccoli with pine nuts, garlic, some of the broccoli cooking water, oil, vinegar, and red pepper until smooth. Serves 4.

Sesame Cauliflower

A rich combination of cauliflower, sesame, tomatoes, and cheese, this goes nicely with soba noodles and a salad.

1 cauliflower, in small chunks, steamed
1 Tbs. olive oil
1 onion, in small chunks
1 lb. tomatoes, in chunks
½ cup mozzarella cheese, grated
½ cup Parmesan cheese, grated
½ cup sesame seeds, toasted

Sauté the onion in olive oil for ten minutes. Add the tomatoes and simmer for fifteen minutes.

Turn into a baking dish with the cauliflower and cheeses. Sprinkle sesame seeds artistically over the top. Bake at 400 degrees for half an hour until the top bubbles to a golden brown. Serves 4.

Lemon Broccoli

This is an easy side dish to serve alongside fish or a casserole.

pot of boiling water
2 lb. broccoli, in spears
2 Tbs. olive oil
splash of lemon juice
sprinkle of lemon zest

Steam the broccoli over boiling water for five minutes. Sauté the steamed broccoli in olive oil for two minutes. Sprinkle with lemon juice, zest, and salt. Serves 4.

Sesame Broccoli

Sesame imparts a smoky, eastern flavor to ordinary broccoli.

1 Tbs. sesame seeds
dash of salt
1 Tbs. olive oil
1 lb. broccoli, in small chunks
2 garlic cloves, crushed
sprinkling of dried red pepper flakes
1 bunch spinach
1 Tbs. sesame oil

Toast sesame seeds in a dry skillet, stirring, until golden. Remove from pan. Cook broccoli, garlic, and red pepper flakes in olive oil for eight minutes. Add spinach and cook another few minutes until spinach wilts. Toss with sesame oil and seeds. Serves 4.

Broccoli Salad

An easy, light side dish. You can add other vegetables and fruits as well—we usually empty the refrigerator into this dish.

pot of boiling water
4 cups broccoli florets or rabe, in small chunks
2 pts. cherry tomatoes, halved
2 tsp. mustard
3 Tbs. rice vinegar
1 Tbs. olive oil
2 Tbs. fresh oregano or 3 tsp. dried oregano

Steam broccoli over pot of water for five minutes. Cool.

Add tomatoes, mustard, vinegar, oil, and oregano. Toss to cover. Chill. Serves 6.

Broccoli Timbale

I adapted this recipe from one by Martha Rose Shulman. There is a lot of dairy in this, so do not eat it often.

pot of boiling water
1 cup broccoli florets
1 cup cauliflower florets
4 eggs
2 cups skim milk
dash of salt, paprika, and pepper
1 cup Parmesan cheese or smoked gouda, grated

Steam the broccoli and cauliflower over boiling water for ten minutes. Chop fine.

In a separate pan, heat the milk until the surface begins to tremble. Remove from heat and beat in the eggs. Stir in the vegetables and other ingredients.

Pour into an oiled 2 quart Bundt pan. Set the pan into a larger pan filled partway with hot water, and place into oven. Bake at 325 degrees for 50 minutes, until beginning to brown. Remove from the oven and cool for ten minutes. Unmold onto a platter. Serves 5.

Broccoli with Peanut Sauce

Reminiscent of our time in Indonesia, this peanut sauce also goes well if you add other vegetables: cauliflower, green beans, and carrots.

5 Tbs. organic peanut butter
4 Tbs. hot water
2 Tbs. soy sauce
2 tsp. Worcestershire sauce
1 clove garlic, crushed
dash of molasses or maple syrup
dash of cayenne
1 lb. broccoli, lightly steamed or raw

Mix the peanut butter, water, soy sauce, Worcestershire sauce, garlic, maple syrup, and cayenne until smooth.

Ladle over raw or cooked broccoli. Toss well. Serves 4.

Cruciferous Vegetable Curry

Eat this for a hefty serving of several cruciferous vegetables. We eat it over brown rice with toasted almonds sprinkled on top for a powerhouse of fertility foods.

1 Tbs. olive oil
1 onion, in small chunks
3 tsp. curry powder
dash of cumin
dash of crushed red pepper
1 cup evaporated skim milk
2 cups potatoes, peeled and in chunks
2 cups tomatoes, in small chunks
3 cups broccoli, in small chunks
1 cup carrots, in small chunks
2 cups cauliflower, in small pieces

Sauté onion in olive oil for five minutes. Add curry, cumin, and red pepper and sauté for another minute. Add milk, potatoes, and the tomatoes. Cover and simmer gently about 20 minutes until the potatoes are tender. Add broccoli, cauliflower and carrots; simmer another ten minutes. Serves 4.

Cauliflower Marranca

Adapted from an old recipe in the original Moosewood cookbook, this is easy to prepare and tasty to eat.

1 onion, in chunks
1 lb. mushrooms, sliced
juice of 1 lemon
1 Tbs. olive oil
1 head cauliflower, in florets
3 cloves garlic, crushed
3 cups brown rice, cooked
2 cups cheddar cheese, grated

Sauté the onion, mushrooms, and lemon in olive oil for ten minutes. Add the cauliflower and garlic, and sauté for a few more minutes.

Place the vegetables, cooked brown rice, and cheese in a casserole dish. Bake uncovered at 350 degrees for 30-40 minutes until it is bubbly on top.

Steamed Cruciferous Heaven

In this dish, broccoli and cauliflower are steamed and mixed with a tomato salad.

pot of boiling water
1 head cauliflower, in small chunks
1 head broccoli, in small chunks
2 carrots, peeled and in chunks
½ lb. olives
3 sun-dried tomatoes, diced
3 Tbs. lemon juice
3 Tbs. olive oil
dash of oregano and dried red pepper

Steam cauliflower, broccoli, and carrots over boiling water until tender, about five minutes. Drain. Add olives and tomatoes.

In a separate bowl, mix lemon juice, oil, and herbs. Pour over vegetables and stir well. Serves 6.

Alfalfa and Leafy Greens

Kale-Apple Salad with Almonds

An exceptionally easy dish to make, the combination of kale and apples is particularly pleasing to the eye and tastebuds. We serve this for company meals with fish and Lime Yams.

¼ cup onion, minced
5 Tbs. apple cider vinegar
2 Tbs. sesame seeds
dash of paprika
2 Tbs. molasses or maple syrup
1/3 cup olive oil
2 Tbs. olive oil
1 cup almonds, slivered
1 bunch of kale, washed and shredded
5 apples, cored and sliced

Mix onion, vinegar, sesame seeds, paprika, most of the molasses, and olive oil together.

Then sauté almonds in olive oil for two minutes. Sprinkle the rest of the molasses into skillet and stir another minute or two. Cool.

Mix kale and apples in a bowl. Toss with dressing, and garnish with almonds. Serves 6.

Arugula Orange Salad

Arugula sets off the sweetness of the orange nicely. You could also substitute collard greens or kale for the arugula.

2 Tbs. olive oil
1 Tbs. balsamic vinegar
½ tsp. orange peel, grated
2 Tbs. orange juice
2 oranges, sectioned and cut into bite-sized chunks
2 endives, separated into leaves
1 bunch arugula, shredded
1 cup walnuts, toasted or plain

Mix the olive oil, vinegar, orange peel and orange juice thoroughly.

Combine orange, endive, and arugula in a bowl, and toss with the dressing. Sprinkle walnuts lavishly on top. Serves 4.

Caramelized Onion Collard Greens

The addition of caramelized onions could make anything taste yummy, and it works particularly well with the slight bitterness of the collard greens. A more elaborate recipe for when you feel like fussing.

2 large onions, cut into small chunks
½ cup olive oil
1 Tbs. molasses
½ cup water or "beef" stock
4 Tbs. balsamic vinegar
6 cups collard greens, shredded
1 cup walnuts, toasted and chopped
1 red onion, thinly sliced

Place two onions onto cookie sheet. Drizzle a bit of the olive oil and the molasses over the top. Bake at 400 degrees for 20 minutes; then turn and bake other side another 20 minutes. Puree with rest of olive oil, water or stock, and vinegar.

Mix the collard greens, walnuts and red onion. Toss with dressing. Serves 6.

Kale & Alfalfa with Mustard Vinaigrette

This yummy dressing also works over collard greens and other leafy green vegetables. For that matter, it also goes well over pasta!

1 Tbs. balsamic vinegar
½ Tbs. lemon juice
1 Tbs. olive oil
2 tsp. mustard
1 bunch of kale, shredded
2 cups alfalfa
1 cup walnuts or almonds

Mix the vinegar, lemon juice, oil and mustard.

In another bowl, combine the kale and alfalfa, Toss with dressing. Sprinkle with walnuts or almonds. Serves 4.

Smoked Salmon, Avocado, and Alfalfa Sandwich

I could not resist including this here, although it is certainly a decadent way to ensure your alfalfa consumption.   This sandwich is lovely for tea parties or luncheons.   It is adapted from a recipe that originally appeared in Gourmet Magazine.

3 Tbs. butter, softened
1 Tbs. lemon juice
½ Tbs. capers
8 slices pumpernickel bread
½ lb. smoked salmon, thinly sliced
1 red onion, thinly sliced
1 avocado, in small chunks
2 cups alfalfa sprouts

Cream together the butter, lemon juice, and capers. Spread on each slice of bread. Layer with the salmon, onion, avocado and sprouts. Makes 4 sandwiches.

Pumpkin and Sunflower Seeds

In addition to the following recipes, pumpkin and sunflower seeds lend themselves to easy eating. Sprinkle a handful over any salad or soup, or simply munch them as snack food. My husband mixes them up with raisins and a very few chocolate chips and is happy for hours.

Pumpkin Seed Brittle

The ultimate in comfort munch food.

1 cup pumpkin seeds
2 Tbs. olive oil
dash of salt
2/3 cup molasses
½ cup water

Toss the pumpkin seeds with olive oil and salt, and place on an ungreased cookie sheet. Bake at 250 degrees, stirring occasionally, for one hour until crisp and golden.

In a skillet, cook the molasses and water over low heat, stirring constantly until it dissolves. Simmer and stir until it turns the color of dark caramels. Stir in the pumpkin seeds. Remove from heat and turn pumpkin seeds onto an oiled sheet of tinfoil, spread thinly. Let cool. Break into pieces. Makes 3 cups.

Seed Focaccia

This is a somewhat complicated recipe, but the results are worth it. The baked focaccia is good hot or cold, and makes great leftover sandwich bread. Thanks to Rochelle Isserow, whose Rosemary Focaccia inspired this recipe.

1 cup warm water
2 Tbs. molasses
2 tsp. dry yeast
4 Tbs. olive oil
1 egg
2 Tbs. butter, melted
dash of salt
5 cups bread flour
1 cup pumpkin seeds
1 cup sunflower seeds

Put warm water, molasses, and yeast in food processor. In about seven minutes, when mixture begins to foam, add 1 Tbs. oil, egg, butter, and salt. Blend. Add flour, pulsing on and off until dough forms and pulls slightly away from the sides. Transfer the dough to a floured surface and knead for a few minutes until smooth. Place into oiled bowl and cover with dry cloth.

Sauté pumpkin seeds and sunflower seeds in remaining olive oil for five minutes, until seeds begin to turn brown. Cool.

Knead the pumpkin seed mixture into the dough.

Divide the dough in two. Press each piece onto an ungreased cookie sheet. Cover loosely and let rise for 40 minutes.

Sprinkle dough with salt and bake at 450 degrees for 15 minutes, until golden brown. Makes 4.

Lace Cookies

The chili and cornmeal give these a southwestern twist, and turn them from dessert cookies into something that goes equally well with a bowl of hearty soup or crock of chili.

¼ cup molasses
2 Tbs. light corn syrup
2 Tbs. butter
2 Tbs. cornmeal
2 Tbs. whole wheat flour
1 tsp. chili powder
¼ cup pumpkin seeds
¼ cup sunflower seeds
2 tsp. lemon juice

Heat molasses, corn syrup, and butter to a boil, stirring constantly. Boil one minute, then remove from heat. Stir in all remaining ingredients. Cool.

With a spoon, scoop dough in blobs onto ungreased cookie sheet. Bake at 350 degrees for ten minutes until golden. Makes 30.

Pumpkin Spice Soup

This is a nice deviation from the standard sweet pumpkin soups. Based on a Mexican recipe, the pumpkin and red pepper give this soup a distinctive zing.

2 Tbs. olive oil
3 cups onion, in small chunks
30 oz. pumpkin puree
1 cup skim milk or cream
dash of dried red pepper
4 cups "beef" stock or water
optional: 1 cup creme fraiche or sour cream
sprinkle of lime juice
1 cup pumpkin seeds, toasted

Sauté the onions in olive oil for ten minutes. Mix in pumpkin, milk and red pepper. Puree. Add stock or water and simmer ten more minutes.

Ladle into bowls, topped with creme fraiche if desired, and a squirt of lime juice. Garnish with pumpkin seeds. Serves 6.

Avocado Seed Salad

This is nice with a big bowl of chili or a curried dish.

3 Tbs. olive oil
3 Tbs. balsamic vinegar
1 Tbs. garlic, crushed
1 head lettuce, Bibb or Boston, shredded
1 bunch of collard greens, steamed
2 avocados, sliced
½ cup pumpkin seeds
½ cup sunflower seeds

Mix olive oil, vinegar, and garlic together.

Toss with lettuce and steamed greens. Garnish with avocado slices and sprinkle with seeds. Serves 6.

Raw Almonds and Walnuts

Raw almonds and walnuts lend themselves to many uses besides those illustrated here. They can be munched whole as snack food; sprinkled into salads and vegetable dishes, and served chopped over desserts. Indeed, the problem with these foods might be the temptation to eat too *much* of them!

Remember that nuts should be stored in the refrigerator, to prevent them from becoming rancid.

Walnut Pepper Pâte

This is a dip for vegetables or pita triangles, that works equally well for company food and family sandwiches.

1 onion, in small chunks
2 garlic cloves, crushed
2 Tbs. olive oil
12 oz. roasted red peppers
1 cup walnuts, toasted
1 Tbs. lemon juice
dash of salt and pepper

Sauté onions and garlic in olive oil for three minutes. Puree remaining ingredients until smooth. Slowly puree in onions and garlic, and the salt and pepper. Serves 2.

Carrot Salad with Nuts

This is a standard carrot salad with a nutty addition that makes it special. Another option is to sprinkle sunflower and pumpkin seeds over the top.

3 Tbs. apple cider vinegar
3 Tbs. honey
dash of salt
½ cup yogurt
4 cups carrots, grated
½ cup raisins
½ cup almonds, toasted and slivered

Mix the vinegar, honey, salt, and yogurt together. Toss with the carrots, raisins, and almonds. Serves 4.

Spicy Nuts

This is another great dish to satisfy the nibbles.   Besides gobbling them down, you can sprinkle spicy nuts over a plain dish of steamed greens for extra flavor.

2 Tbs. olive oil
dash of cayenne, cumin, and salt
3 cups walnuts
2 cups almonds

Sauté the spices in olive oil, stirring constantly for one minute. Add the nuts and coat thoroughly.

Place the walnuts and almonds in a pan and bake at 350 degrees for ten minutes. Cool. Makes 5 cups.

Baked Apricot Pie

This is a simple dish that is elegant simply because it is rare to see an apricot pie. The apricots combine well with the nuts.

1 9-inch pie crust
¼ cup apricot preserves
1 cup almonds, pureed
10 apricots, halved
3 Tbs. maple syrup

Spread apricot preserves evenly in the bottom of a pie crust. Layer almonds on top. Arrange apricots on top of the almonds. Drizzle maple syrup on top. Bake at 400 degrees for one hour. Serves 6.

Sweet and Spicy Nuts

I designed these after tasting the snackfood MeshugaNuts, which are probably made with meringue. This version is butter and egg-free.

½ cup maple syrup
4 cups almonds
1 Tbs. pepper
dash of salt

In a saucepan, heat the maple syrup. Add almonds and toss until covered. Cook over medium heat for five minutes until syrup thickens, stirring often.   Sprinkle salt and pepper into mixture.

Transfer almonds to an ungreased baking sheet.   Bake at 200 degrees for ten minutes, until golden.   Store in canister. Makes 4 cups.

Wheat Germ

As with nuts and seeds, wheat germ is something that lends itself to a great variety of foods. In addition to the following recipes provided here, try sprinkling wheat germ on top of your breakfast grain or cereal in the morning. Add it to a pita and vegetable sandwich for lunch. Or stir it into your soup or curry for dinner. Wheat germ even provides a nice crunchy topping for fruit, cake, even ice cream. After a while, wheat germ will be so much a part of your diet, you may have to do what we did, and put it into its own shaker on the table, right beside the salt.

Remember to store your wheat germ in the refrigerator to prevent the oils from becoming rancid.

Banana Wheat Germ Muffins

Muffins are an easy way to incorporate your day's allotment of wheat germ, and a delectable one at that. This recipe calls for bananas, but you can substitute almost any fruit to make these yummy muffins.

2 cups whole wheat flour
¾ cup molasses
1 Tbs. baking powder
¾ tsp. salt
1 cup wheat germ, toasted
3 bananas, mashed
½ cup milk
2 eggs
1/3 cup vegetable oil
1 tsp. vanilla extract

Stir flour, molasses, baking powder salt and wheat germ together. Add bananas, milk, eggs, oil, and vanilla and stir until batter is just moistened. Divide into twelve muffin cups.

Bake at 350 degrees for 20 minutes or until golden brown. Makes a dozen.

Wheat Germ Pancakes

We make up a big batch of this batter each week and keep it in the refrigerator, so that we can whip up hot pancakes each morning with little hassle.

1 cup whole wheat flour
1 tsp. baking soda
dash of salt
dash of sugar
½ cup wheat germ
1 egg
1 cup buttermilk
½ cup walnuts

Mix the flour, baking soda, salt, sugar, wheat germ, egg and buttermilk in a blender.   Add in the walnuts and blend until walnuts are very fine.

Pour by teaspoon onto hot oiled griddle, and cook for one minute on each side, until golden. Makes 3 dozen.

Granola

The best thing about granola (besides its crunchy yummy taste) is that it is very forgiving. Add whatever you want to this one—just be sure that you leave in the wheat germ! The nuts and seeds in this version are an added bonus.

1 cup oats
1 cup wheat germ
1 cup sesame seeds
1 cup sunflower seeds
1 cup almonds
1 cup walnuts
1 cup maple syrup
½ cup sesame oil
½ cup water
splash of vanilla extract
1 cup raisins
1 cup dates, in small chunks

Mix the dry ingredients together in a bowl. Add in the liquid ingredients, stirring to moisten everything.

Oil a few cookie trays. Scoop the granola onto the trays and bake at 250 degrees for one hour, stirring every ten minutes so it does not burn. After baking, immediately mix in the dried fruit. Makes lots.

Wheat Germ Cereal with Yogurt

This is a variation of Birchermuesli, a breakfast staple in many countries.

1 cup oats
1 cup wheat germ
3 cups yogurt
½ cup raisins
½ cup dates
½ cup apples, in small chunks
½ cup almonds, toasted
½ cup walnuts, toasted
2 Tbs. honey
2 Tbs. lemon juice

Combine all the ingredients until well blended. Refrigerate one hour. Serves 4.

Appendix A:
Other Things to Try

This appendix includes other ideas and suggestions of things to try that may promote fertility. Most of these items are anecdotal, and have not been studied scientifically or systematically. Of course, there are also people who swear they work. In general, these suggestions are probably less likely to affect your fertility and ability to carry to term than the nutritional and lifestyle points detailed earlier in the book; however, in the interest of thoroughness they are included, and none of them are likely to be harmful.

Use gravity: Anecdotes abound of women who stood on their head after intercourse, or elevated their hips, and were able to conceive. One scientist suggests that perhaps gravity assists in pulling the sperm down to the egg. (The other opinion is that regardless of your position, sperm will swim up through cervical fluid.) A tip more likely to help is to have intercourse in the missionary position (man on top) as this will ensure that sperm are deposited closer to the cervix.

Incorporate a waiting period: Try abstaining from intercourse for several days after menstruation ends. It is believed that this abstinence might increase the sperm count. (Of course, if you ovulate early, such a waiting period could be equally likely to cause you to miss your fertile period altogether.) See the earlier discussion on pinpointing your ovulation before trying this one.

Try cough syrup: Some women use Robitussin or other cough syrups to thin cervical fluid; the ostensible reason this works is that it serves to lessen the barrier effect of the cervical fluid. Try 2 teaspoons (orally) three times a day with a glass of water, for the five consecutive days before ovulation begins. Be certain, however, to avoid cough remedies that contain antihistamines, as these may dry up your cervical fluid completely, rendering fertilization highly unlikely, (because the sperm require a certain amount of cervical fluid in which to swim.)

Try baking soda: Some anecdotal evidence suggests that women can somewhat counteract the effects of low sperm count of their mate by consuming baking soda, as this will decrease vaginal acidity (and presumably thereby allow more sperm to survive). Try a teaspoon twice a day, the amount recommended for indigestion.

Avoid heat, tight pants & bicycles: Both men and women should stay away from saunas, electric blankets, and really hot baths. One study also pointed to the popularity of tight-fitting underwear as a possible cause in lowered sperm count; it is speculated that if the scrotal sac becomes too warm, it might result in lethargic sperm. Men should also avoid riding bicycles, because the friction and resulting heat might have the same effect. A later study has cast this theory into doubt; still, like everything else in this book, it can't hurt.

Sniff a baby: Anecdotes claim that if you have a hormonal problem impeding fertility, holding a baby will help. The medical explanation might be that the pheromones in the sweat have some effect; theoretically, the sweat of a pregnant women should be similarly effective.

Avoid environmental contaminants: A strong argument can be made for the negative role of environmental pollutants on fertility and miscarriage rates. Studies have made the link with everything from polychlorobiphenyls (PCBs) on miscarriage rates to pesticides on fertility. A 1998 article in a leading

French fertility journal suggested a strong relationship between environmental conditions and spermatogenesis, citing both dibromochloropropane distilbenes and gossypol as recent culprits implicated in fertility studies. Chlordane, a pesticide found in the air of 75% of United States homes, has also been implicated in infertility, according to an article in *Teratogenesis, Carcinogenesis, Mutagenesis.* Hair spray, nail polish remover, and dry cleaning have all been implicated. And inhalation of car exhaust is now thought to decrease fertility, according to a 1995 *Environmental Health Perspectives* study.

Try herbs: Certain herbs are used extensively in other cultures to promote fertility. Well-known herbalist Susun Weed recommends dried red clover flower, nettle leaves, and red raspberry leaves. For more information on herbal solutions to infertility, see her book, *Wise Woman Herbal for the Childbearing Year*, pages 2-3.

Go on vacation! In the same way that relaxation, meditation, and yoga can help in promoting fertility, many people claim that the stress reduction involved in vacationing helped them to conceive. And remember that a deficiency of vitamin D in animals discouraged fertility—and that the best way to increase your vitamin D levels is by going out in the sun!

Appendix B:
Sources of Nutrients

Nutrient	Source
Vitamin A	cruciferous vegetables, alfalfa
Arginine	nuts
Beta Carotene	yams
Vitamin B2 (Riboflavin)	almonds, wheat germ

Vitamin B6 (Pyridoxine)	soy, wheat germ, whole grains, walnuts, sunflower seeds
Bioflavonoids	cruciferous vegetables
Vitamin C	cruciferous vegetables, alfalfa
Calcium	soy, broccoli, alfalfa
Chromium	whole grains
Vitamin D	alfalfa
Vitamin E	whole grains, broccoli, alfalfa, nuts, wheat germ, seeds, leafy greens, soy
Folic Acid	leafy greens, whole grains, wheat germ, soy,
Indoles	cruciferous vegetables
Iron	alfalfa, leafy greens
Vitamin K	alfalfa, leafy greens, soy

Magnesium	alfalfa, whole grains, leafy greens, nuts
PABA	wheat germ, leafy greens
Phosphorous	alfalfa, nuts
Selenium	wheat germ, garlic, whole grains, sunflower seeds,
Sulforaphane	cruciferous vegetables
Zinc	wheat germ, seeds, soy

Bibliography:
For More Information

Resolve is a national infertility support organization offering support, education, and advocacy to those experiencing infertility. Their services include a national Help Line, quarterly newsletter, literature list, and local support groups through over 50 chapters. Contact them for information on support groups in your area. Resolve, 1310 Broadway, Somerville, MA 02144-1731, (617) 623-0744.

Infertility Awareness Association of Canada, 774 Echo Drive, Suite 523, Ottawa, Ontario K1S 5N8, Canada (613)730-1322; (800)263-2929 in Canada

Endometriosis Association Education Support Research, 8585 North 76th Place, Milwaukee, WI 53223. (414)355-2200.

Articles:

Of the several hundred medical studies I examined to research this book, these are the ones I recommend as most salient.

Abdel Aziz AH, Shouman SA, Attia AS, Saad SF
A study on the reproductive toxicity of erythrosine in male mice. *Pharmacol Res* (1997);35(5):457-62.

Abraham G
Nutritional factors in the etiology of the premenstrual tension syndromes. *J Reprod Med* (1983)28:452.

Akingbemi BT, Rao PV, Aire TA
Chronic ethanol intake may delay the onset of gossypol-induced infertility in the male rat. *Andrologia* (1997);29(4):201-7.

Bahamondes L, Saboya W, Tambascia M, Trevisan M
Galactorrhea, infertility, and short luteal phases in hyperprolactinemic women: Early stages of amenorrhea-galactorrhea? *Fert Steril* (1979)32:476.

Baird D
Smokers face higher infertility. *Journal of American Medical Association* (1985);253:2979-83.

Beerendonk CC, Derkx FH, Schellekens AP, Hop WC, van Dop PA
The influence of dietary sodium restriction on renal and ovarian renin and prorenin production during ovarian stimulation. *Hum Reprod* (1996);11(5):956-61.

Blanchard T, Ferguson J, Love L, Takeda T, Henderson B, Hasler J, Chalup W
Effect of dietary crude-protein type on fertilization and embryo quality in dairy cattle. *Am J Vet Res.* (1990):51(6):905-8

Bolumar F, Olsen J, Rebagliato M, Bisanti L
Caffeine intake and delayed conception: a European multicenter study on infertility and subfecundity. *Am J Epidemiol* (1997);145(4):324-34.

Bujan L
Environment and spermatogenesis. *Contracept Fertil Sex* (1998);26(1):39-48.

Burger, Henry G
Neuroendocrine control of human ovulation. *International Journal of Fertility* (1981); 26:153-60

Check, Jerome H
Comparison of various therapies for the luteinized unruptured follicle syndrome. *International Journal of Fertility* (1992):37:33-40

Clark AM, Thornley B, Tomlinson L, Galletley C, Norman RJ
Weight loss in obese infertile women results in improvement in reproductive outcome for all forms of fertility treatment. *Hum Reprod* (1998):13(6):1502-5

Chowaniec T, Lorenz K, Guzikowski W
Concentration of some trace elements in the semen of men. *Ginekol Pol* (1989):60(4):223-8

Corenblum B, Pairaudeau N, Shewchuk A
Prolactin hypersecretion and short luteal phase defects. *Obstet Gynecol* (1976)47:487.

Cramer DW, Xu H, Sahi T
Adult hypolactasia, milk consumption, and age-specific fertility. *Am J Epidemiol* (1994);139(3):282-9.

Dabrowski K, Ciereszko A
Ascorbic acid protects against male infertility in a teleost fish. *Experientia* (1996);52(2):97-100.

Daly Douglas
Ultrasonographic assessment of luteinized unruptured follicle syndrome in unexplained infertility.   *Fertility and Sterility* (1985) 43: 62-5

Damir HA, Barri ME, el Hassan SM, Tageldin MH, Wahbi AA, Idris OF
Clinical zinc and copper deficiencies in cattle of western Sudan. *Trop Anim Health Prod* (1988):20(1):52-6

Darland Nancy
Infertility associated with luteal phase defect.   *Journal of Obstetric, Gynecologic and Neonatal Nursing* (1985): 212-7

Dawson EB, Harris WA, Powell LC
Relationship between ascorbic acid and male fertility.   *World Rev Nutr Diet.* (1990): 62:2-26.

Dennefors B, Sjogren A, Hamberger L
Progesterone and adenosine 3',5'-monophosphate formation by isolated human corpora lutea of different ages: Influence of human chorionic gonadotropin and prostaglandins. *J Clin Endocrinol Metab* (1982)55:102.

Dickman MD, Leung CK, Leong MK
Hong Kong male subfertility links to mercury in human hair and fish. *Sci Total Environ* (1998);214:165-74.

Favier A
Current aspects about the role of zinc in nutrition. *Rev Prat* (1993);43(2):146-51.

Ferguson JD, Blanchard T, Galligan DT, Hoshall DC, Chalupa W
Infertility in dairy cattle fed a high percentage of protein degradable in the rumen. *J Am Vet Med Assoc* (1988):192(5):659-62.

Fish L, Mariash C
Hyperprolactinemia, Infertility, and Hypothyroidism. *Archives of Internal Medicine* (1988) 148:709-11

France J
Overview of the biological aspects of the female period. *International Journal of Fertility* (1981) 26: 143-52

Franks S, Robinson S, Willis DS
Nutrition, insulin and polycystic ovary syndrome. *Rev Reprod* (1996);1(1):47-53.

Frisch R
Fatness and fertility. *Sci Am* (1988)92

Furuhjelm M, Jonson B
Miscarriage more common with low sperm counts. *International J of Fertility* (1962);7(1):17-21.

Goldenberg R, White R
The effect of vaginal lubricants on sperm motility in vitro. *Fertility and Sterility* (1975)26:872-3.

Goldin B, Adlercreutz H, Gorbach S, Warram J, Dwyer J, Swenson L, Woods M
Estrogen excretion patterns and plasma levels in vegetarian and omnivorous women. *New England Journal of Medicine* (1982)307:1542.

Grodstein F
Relation of female infertility to consumption of caffeinated beverages. *American Journal of Epidemiology.* (1993)137:1353-9.

Gui-Yuan Z, Meng-Chun J, Jin-Lai C, Wen-Qing Y
The effect of long-term treatment with crude cotton seed oil on pituitary and testicular function in men. *Int J Androl* (1989):12(6):404-10

Hargrove J, Abraham G
Effect of vitamin B6 on infertility in women with the premenstrual tension syndrome. *Infertility* (1979)2:315.

Hargrove J, Abraham G
Abnormal luteal function in women with endometriosis. *Fertil Steril* (1983)34:302.

Hartoma T, Nahoul K, Netter A
Zinc, plasma androgens and male sterility. *Lancet* (1977) 1125-6.

Hirsch KS, Adams ER, Hoffman DG, Markham JK, Owen NV
Studies to elucidate the mechanism of fenarimol-induced infertility in male rats. *Toxicol Appl Pharmacol* (1986):86(3):391-9.

Horrobin D
The role of essential fatty acids and prostaglandins in the premenstrual syndrome. *J Reprod Med* (1983) 28:465.

Ibeh IN, Uraih N, Ogonar JI
Dietary exposure to aflatoxin in human male infertility in Benin City, Nigeria. *Int J Fertil Menopausal Stud* (1994);39(4):208-14.

Igiene C
PCB and other organochlorine compounds in blood of women with or without miscarriage: a hypothesis of correlation. *Ecotoxicol Environ Saf* (1989):17(1):1-11

Ingraham RH, Kappel LC, Morgan EB, Srikandakumar A
Correction of subnormal fertility with copper and magnesium supplementation. *J Dairy Sci* (1987):70(1):167-80

Inpanbutr N, Reiswig JD, Bacon WL, Slemons RD, Iacopino AM
Effect of vitamin D on testicular CaBP28K expression and serum testosterone in chicken. *Biol Reprod* (1996); 54(1):242-8.

Isong EU, Ebong PE, Ifon ET, Umoh IB, Eka OU
Thermoxidized palm oil induces reproductive toxicity in healthy and malnourished rats. *Plant Foods Hum Nutr* (1997);51(2):159-66.

Jameson S
Zinc status in pregnancy: the effect of zinc therapy on perinatal mortality, prematurity, and placental ablation. *Ann NY Acad Sci* (1993);678:178-92.

Jones H, Toner J
The infertile couple. *New England Journal of Medicine.* (1993)7: 1710-5.

Kalra SP, Kalra PS
Nutritional infertility: the role of the interconnected hypothalamic neuropeptide Y-galanin-opioid network. *Front Neuroendocrinol* (1996);17(4):371-401.

Kauppila A, Leinonen P, Vihko R, "Ylostalo P
Metoclopramide-induced hyperprolactinemia impairs ovarian follicle maturation and corpus luteum function in women. *J Clin Endocrinol Metab.* (1982)54:955.

Kutteh WH, Chao CH, Ritter JO, Byrd W
Vaginal lubricants for the infertile couple: effect on sperm activity. *Int J Fertil Menopausal Stud* (1996);41(4):400-4.

Lenton E, Landgren B, Sexton L
Normal variation in the length of the luteal phase of the menstrual cycle: Identification of the short luteal phase. *British Journal of Obstetrics and Gynecology* (1984) 91: 685-9.

Luke B
Nutrition during pregnancy. *Curr Opin Obstet Gynecol* (1994);6(5):402-7.

Matossian MK
Fertility decline in Europe, 1875-1913. Was zinc deficiency the cause? *Perspect Biol Med* (1991): 34(4):604-16.

Monsees TK, Winterstein U, Schill WB, Miska W
Influence of gossypol on the secretory function of cultured rat sertoli cells. *Toxicon* (1998):36(5):813-6

Murill WB
Prepubertal genistein exposure suppresses mammary cancer and enhances gland differentiation in rats. *Carcinogenesis* (1996); 17(77):1451-7.

Ondrizek RR, Chan PJ, Patton WC, King A
An alternative medicine study of herbal effects on the penetration of zona-free hamster oocytes and the integrity of sperm deoxyribonucleic acid. *Fertility and Sterility* (1999);71(3):517-522.

Olney JW
MSG increases odds of infertility and obesity - shorter growth. *Science* (1969);164:719-721.

Olsen J
Cigarette smoking, tea and coffee drinking, and subfecundity. *American Journal of Epidemiology* (1991)133(7):734-9.

Osweiler GD, Stahr HM, Beran GW
Relationship of mycotoxins to swine reproductive failure. *J Vet Diagn Invest* (1990):2(1):73-5

Padilla S, Craft K
Anovulation: Etiology, evaluation and management. *Nurse Practitioner* (1985)10(12):28-44.

Pirke KM, Schweiger U, Laessie R, Dickhaut B, Schweiger M, Waechtler M
Dieting influences the menstrual cycle: vegetarian versus nonvegetarian diet. *Fertil Steril* (1986):46(6):1083-8.

Prasad A
Clinical, endocrinologic and biochemical effects of zinc deficiency. *Spec Topics in Endocrinol Metab* (1985)7:59-60.

Ravnskov U
Do polyunsaturated fats cause male sterility? *Lakartidningen* (1994);91(23):2308

Rayman MP
Dietary selenium: time to act. *BMJ* (1997);314(7078):387-8.

Schlegel P, Chang T, Marshall G
Antibiotics: Potential hazards to male fertility. *Fertility and Sterility* (1991)55:235-242.

Scott R, MacPherson A, Yates RW, Hussain B, Dixon J
The effect of oral selenium supplementation on human sperm motility. *Br J Urol* (1998):82(1):76-80.

Seppala M, Hirvonen E, Ranta T
Hyperprolactinaemia and luteal insufficiency. *Lancet* (1976)229

Setchell KD, Gosselin SJ, Welsh MB, Johnston JO, Balistreri WF, Kramer LW, Dresser BL, Tarr MJ
Dietary estrogens—a probable cause of infertility and liver disease in captive cheetahs. *Gastroenterology* (1987):93(2):225-33.

Simha R.
Post-testicular antifertility effects of Abrus precatorius seed extract in albino rats. *J Ethnopharmacol.* (1990):28(2): 173-81.

Smith S
The short luteal phase and infertility. *British Journal of Obstetrics and Gynecology* (1984) 91:1120-2.

Souka A
Effect of aspirin on the luteal phase of human menstrual cycle. *Contraception.* (1984) 29:181-8.

Steward DE. Robinson E, Goldbloom DS, Wright C
Infertility and eating disorders. *Am J. Obstet Gynecol.* (1990):1196-9.

Thomas R, Reid R
Thyroid disease and reproductive dysfunction: A review. *Obstetrics & Gynecology* (1987)70:789-92.

Umapathy E
Antifertility effects of cowpeas on male rats. *Cent Afr J Med* (1993);39(3):52-6.

Verma SP
Curcumin and genistein, plant natural products show synergistic inhibiting effects on the growth of human breast cancer MCF-7 cells induced by estrogenic pesticides. *Biochemical and Biophysical Communications* (1997);233:692-6.

Wade GN, Schneider JE, Li HY
Control of fertility by metabolic cues. *Am J Physiol* (1996);270(1):E1-19.

Wang XG
Teratogenic effect of potato glycoalkaloids. *Chung Hua Fu Chan Ko Tsa Chih* (1993);28(2):73-5, 121-2.

Weathersbee P, Lodge J
Caffeine: Its direct and indirect influence on reproduction. *J Reprod Med* (1977)19:60.

Wilcox AJ, Weinberg CR, Baird DD
Timing of sexual intercourse in relation to ovulation—effects on the probability of conception, survival of the pregnancy, and sex of the baby. *The New England Journal of Medicine* (1995):333(23):1517-21.

Wu S, Oldfield J, Whanger P, Weswig P
Effect of selenium, vitamin E, and antioxidants on testicular function in rats. *Biol Reprod* (1973)8:625.

Wynn A
Nutrition before conception and the outcome of pregnancy. *Nutr Health* (1987):5(1-2):31-43

Wynn A, Wynn M
Magnesium and other nutrient deficiencies as possible causes of hypertension and low birthweight. *Nutr Health.* (1988):6(2):69-88.

Glossary

Anovulation: The absence of ovulation.

ART (assisted reproductive technology): All treatments or procedures that involve the handling of human eggs and sperm for the purpose of establishing a pregnancy. Types of ART include IVF (in vitro fertilization), GIFT (gamete intrafallopian transfer), ZIFT (zygote intrafallopian transfer), embryo cryopreservation, egg or embryo donation, and surrogate birth.

Cervical Fluid: The secretion produced in the cervix that acts as an alkaline medium to protect sperm in the acidic conditions of the vagina. A woman typically produces cervical fluid only in the days before ovulation.   Slippery, eggwhite-like cervical fluid is most fertile.

Cervix: The lower part of the uterus that projects into the vagina.

Clomid: (Clomiphene Citrate) A drug commonly used to induce ovulation.

Corpus Luteum: The remains of the ruptured follicle after ovulation.   In the absence of a pregnancy, the corpus luteum disintegrates within 12 to 16 days.   If the egg is fertilized, the corpus luteum produces progesterone to support the early pregnancy until the placenta forms.

Egg: A female reproductive cell, also called an oocyte or ovum.

Egg transfer: The transfer of retrieved eggs into a woman's fallopian tubes through laparoscopy, used only in GIFT (gamete intrafallopian transfer).

Embryo: The initial stages of development of an egg that has been fertilized by a sperm and has undergone one or more divisions to six weeks after conception.

Endocrinologist: A doctor specializing in the function of hormones.

Endometriosis: The presence of tissue similar to the uterine lining in locations outside of the uterus, such as the ovaries, fallopian tubes, and abdominal cavity. Endometriosis may cause infertility.

Endometrium: The lining of the uterus which is shed during menstruation. With conception, the fertilized egg implants in the endometrium.

Estrogen: The hormone produced in the ovaries, responsible for controlling the menstrual cycle. Increasing estrogen levels cause fertile cervical fluid.

Fallopian tube: A tube through which the mature egg tumbles from the ovary toward the uterus. Sperm swim from the uterus toward the fallopian tube, where fertilization may take place.

Fertilization: Penetration of the egg by the sperm and the resulting fusion of genetic material that develops into an embryo.

Fetus: A developing embryo from six weeks after fertilization until birth.

Follicle: A fluid-filled structure in the ovary containing the egg. At ovulation, the follicle ruptures the surface of the ovary, releasing the egg.

Follicle Stimulating Hormone: The hormone produced by the pituitary gland that stimulates the ovaries to produce the hormone estrogen.

Gamete: A reproductive cell, either a sperm or an egg.

GIFT (gamete intrafallopian transfer): An ART procedure that involves removing eggs from the woman's ovary, combining them with sperm, and using laparoscopy to place the unfertilized eggs and the sperm into the woman's fallopian tubes through a small abdominal incision. As distinct from IVF, the actual fertilization takes place in the fallopian tube, rather than a laboratory.

Gonadotropin Releasing Hormone (GNRH): A chemical substance produced by the brain's hypothalamus, it stimulates the pituitary gland to produce first follicle stimulating hormone and then luteinizing hormone, leading respectively to follicular development and ovulation.

Gonadotropins: Hormones produced by the pituitary gland, including follicle stimulating hormone and luteinizing hormone.

Human Chorionic Gonadotropin (HCG): A pregnancy hormone produced by the developing embryo at implantation into the uterine lining. HCG maintains the corpus luteum and secretion of progesterone until the placenta develops.

Intra-Uterine Insemination (IUI):   A medical procedure in which sperm are inserted via catheter through the cervix directly into the uterus.

IVF (in vitro fertilization):   An ART procedure that involves removing eggs from the woman's ovaries and fertilizing them with sperm outside her body in a laboratory. Two days later the resulting embryos are transferred into the woman's uterus through the cervix.

Laparoscopy: A surgical procedure in which a laparoscope (a fiber-optic instrument) is inserted into the pelvic area through a small abdominal incision.

Luteal Phase: The latter part of the cycle from ovulation to the beginning of the next menstruation. This phase can last between 12 to 16 days, but within individuals rarely varies in length.

Luteinizing Hormone: The hormone produced by the pituitary gland that is released in a surge, causing ovulation.

Oocyte: Female reproductive cell; egg, ovum.

Ovulation: The release of a mature egg from the ovarian follicle.

Pituitary Gland: The gland responsible for hormonal control of the ovaries and testes.

Progesterone: A hormone produced by the corpus luteum in the ovary after ovulation occurs. It prepares the endometrium for possible pregnancy.

Sperm Count: A calculation of the total number of sperm, as well as their morphology (shape and size) and motility (forward moving ability).

Subfertility: Below average fertility.

ZIFT (zygote intrafallopian transfer): An ART procedure in which eggs are collected from a woman's ovary and fertilized in a laboratory. Laparoscopy is then used to place the resulting fertilized egg, or zygote, into the woman's fallopian tubes through a small abdominal incision.

Zygote: A fertilized egg, immediately after fertilization. (After further cell division, this becomes an embryo.)

Index

B

C

D

H

O

P

T

U

V

W

Menu Planner

Your Menu:

    Breakfast:
    Lunch:
    Snack:
    Dinner:

Food Categories Covered:

Category:	**Dish:**
Yams:	
Garlic:	
Tofu & Black Soybeans:	
Kelp:	
Whole Grains:	
Cruciferous Vegetables:	
Alfalfa & Leafy Greens:	
Pumpkin & Sunflower Seeds:	
Almonds and Walnuts:	
Wheat Germ:	

Menu Planner

Your Menu:

      Breakfast:
      Lunch:
      Snack:
      Dinner:

Food Categories Covered:

Category:	**Dish:**
Yams:	
Garlic:	
Tofu & Black Soybeans:	
Kelp:	
Whole Grains:	
Cruciferous Vegetables:	
Alfalfa & Leafy Greens:	
Pumpkin & Sunflower Seeds:	
Almonds and Walnuts:	
Wheat Germ:	

Menu Planner

Your Menu:
    Breakfast:
    Lunch:
    Snack:
    Dinner:

Food Categories Covered:

Category:	**Dish:**
Yams:	
Garlic:	
Tofu & Black Soybeans:	
Kelp:	
Whole Grains:	
Cruciferous Vegetables:	
Alfalfa & Leafy Greens:	
Pumpkin & Sunflower Seeds:	
Almonds and Walnuts:	
Wheat Germ:	

Menu Planner

Your Menu:

   Breakfast:
   Lunch:
   Snack:
   Dinner:

Food Categories Covered:

Category:	**Dish:**
Yams:	
Garlic:	
Tofu & Black Soybeans:	
Kelp:	
Whole Grains:	
Cruciferous Vegetables:	
Alfalfa & Leafy Greens:	
Pumpkin & Sunflower Seeds:	
Almonds and Walnuts:	
Wheat Germ:	

Menu Planner

Your Menu:

    Breakfast:
    Lunch:
    Snack:
    Dinner:

Food Categories Covered:

Category:	**Dish:**
Yams:	
Garlic:	
Tofu & Black Soybeans:	
Kelp:	
Whole Grains:	
Cruciferous Vegetables:	
Alfalfa & Leafy Greens:	
Pumpkin & Sunflower Seeds:	
Almonds and Walnuts:	
Wheat Germ:	

Menu Planner

Your Menu:
>Breakfast:
>Lunch:
>Snack:
>Dinner:

Food Categories Covered:

Category:	**Dish:**
Yams:	
Garlic:	
Tofu & Black Soybeans:	
Kelp:	
Whole Grains:	
Cruciferous Vegetables:	
Alfalfa & Leafy Greens:	
Pumpkin & Sunflower Seeds:	
Almonds and Walnuts:	
Wheat Germ:	

Menu Planner

Your Menu:
- Breakfast:
- Lunch:
- Snack:
- Dinner:

Food Categories Covered:

Category:	**Dish:**
Yams:	
Garlic:	
Tofu & Black Soybeans:	
Kelp:	
Whole Grains:	
Cruciferous Vegetables:	
Alfalfa & Leafy Greens:	
Pumpkin & Sunflower Seeds:	
Almonds and Walnuts:	
Wheat Germ:	

Menu Planner

Your Menu:
    Breakfast:
    Lunch:
    Snack:
    Dinner:

Food Categories Covered:

Category:	**Dish:**
Yams:	
Garlic:	
Tofu & Black Soybeans:	
Kelp:	
Whole Grains:	
Cruciferous Vegetables:	
Alfalfa & Leafy Greens:	
Pumpkin & Sunflower Seeds:	
Almonds and Walnuts:	
Wheat Germ:	

Menu Planner

Your Menu:
    Breakfast:
    Lunch:
    Snack:
    Dinner:

Food Categories Covered:

Category:	**Dish:**
Yams:	
Garlic:	
Tofu & Black Soybeans:	
Kelp:	
Whole Grains:	
Cruciferous Vegetables:	
Alfalfa & Leafy Greens:	
Pumpkin & Sunflower Seeds:	
Almonds and Walnuts:	
Wheat Germ:	

Fern Reiss is a widely published author. She studied nutrition and cooking at the Kushi Institute for Macrobiotic Studies in Massachusetts and the Culinary Institute of America in New York, and is a member of the American Culinary Federation. She lives with her husband and two children in Boston.

A nutrition and fertility expert on the radio and talk show circuit, she also gives intensive seminars on **The Infertility Diet** across the country. To receive information on her seminar schedule, or inquire about booking her for seminars or speaking engagements, email her publisher at info@infertilitydiet.com, or send a self-addressed, stamped envelope to:

Peanut Butter and Jelly Press
P.O. Box 239
Newton Center, MA 02459-0002

Please send ____ copies of **The Infertility Diet**, at $24.95 each. In Massachusetts, add 5% sales tax ($1.25 per book). Shipping: $3.20 for first book ordered; $1 for each additional book. All books are shipped priority mail, discreetly wrapped.

____I'm not ordering now, but please add me to your mailing list for infertility/miscarriage nutritional updates and related information.

Name:
Address:
City: State:
Zip:
telephone: (   )
email:
circle one: VISA   MasterCard
Card Number: Expires:

Peanut Butter and Jelly Press
P.O. Box 239
Newton, MA 02459-0002
phone/fax: (617)630-0945; (800)408-6226
www.infertilitydiet.com   info@infertilitydiet.com